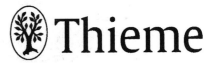

Split Cord Malformations

Ashok K. Mahapatra, MS, MCh, DNB, MAMS, FNAS
Vice-Chancellor
Siksha 'O' Anusandhan University
Bhubaneshwar, Odisha
Former Chief of Neurosciences Center
Former Head of Department of Neurosurgery
All India Institute of Medical Sciences
New Delhi, India

Sachin A. Borkar, MCh, FACS, DNB, MNAMS
Additional Professor
Department of Neurosurgery
All India Institute of Medical Sciences
New Delhi, India

Subhashree Mahapatra, BSc, MSc, PhD
Development Manager
Asia Pacific Region
Lipotec Ltd.
New Delhi, India

Thieme
Delhi • Stuttgart • New York • Rio de Janeiro

Publishing Director: Ritu Sharma
Development Editor: Dr Gurvinder Kaur
Director-Editorial Services: Rachna Sinha
Project Manager: Gaurav Prabhu
Vice President, Sales and Marketing:
Arun Kumar Majji
Managing Director & CEO: Ajit Kohli

Thieme Medical and Scientific Publishers Private
Limited.
A - 12, Second Floor, Sector - 2, Noida - 201 301,
Uttar Pradesh, India, +911204556600
Email: customerservice@thieme.in
www.thieme.in

Cover design: Thieme Publishing Group
Typesetting by RECTO Graphics, India

Printed in India by Nutech Print Services

5 4 3 2 1

ISBN: 978-81-948570-9-9

Important note: Medicine is an ever-changing science undergoing continual development. Research and clinical experience are continually expanding our knowledge, in particular, our knowledge of proper treatment and drug therapy. Insofar as this book mentions any dosage or application, readers may rest assured that the authors, editors, and publishers have made every effort to ensure that such references are in accordance with **the state of knowledge at the time of production of the book.**

Nevertheless, this does not involve, imply, or express any guarantee or responsibility on the part of the publishers in respect to any dosage instructions and forms of applications stated in the book. **Every user is requested to examine carefully** the manufacturers' leaflets accompanying each drug and to check, if necessary, in consultation with a physician or specialist, whether the dosage schedules mentioned therein or the contraindications stated by the manufacturers differ from the statements made in the present book. Such examination is particularly important with drugs that are either rarely used or have been newly released in the market. Every dosage schedule or every form of application used is entirely at the user's own risk and responsibility. The authors and publishers request every user to report to the publishers any discrepancies or inaccuracies noticed. If errors in this work are found after publication, errata will be posted at www.thieme.com on the product description page.

Some of the product names, patents, and registered designs referred to in this book are in fact registered trademarks or proprietary names even though specific reference to this fact is not always made in the text. Therefore, the appearance of a name without designation as proprietary is not to be construed as a representation by the publisher that it is in the public domain.

Contents

Preface   vii

About the Authors   ix

Contributors   xi

1. Introduction to Split Cord Malformations   1
   Amol Raheja, Sanjeev A. Sreenivasan, and Ashok K. Mahapatra

2. Embryology of Split Cord Malformations   7
   Ashutosh Agarwal, Shweta Kedia, and Ashok K. Mahapatra

3. Classification of Split Cord Malformations   15
   Dattaraj P. Sawarkar, Deepak K. Gupta, and Ashok K. Mahapatra

4. Split Cord Malformations Type I   29
   Shweta Kedia, Rajesh Meena, and Ashok K. Mahapatra

5. Split Cord Malformations Type II   41
   Amol Raheja, Tarang K. Vora, and Ashok K. Mahapatra

6. Dorsal Spur   51
   Sachin A. Borkar, Mohit Agrawal, and Ashok K. Mahapatra

7. Cervical Split Cord Malformations   61
   Sachin A. Borkar, Ravi Sreenivasan, and Ashok K. Mahapatra

8. Composite Split Cord Malformations or Multisite Split Cord Malformations   79
   Kanwaljeet Garg, Hitesh Inder Singh Rai, and Pankaj K. Singh

9. Adult Split Cord Malformations   89
   Mohit Agrawal, Manoj Phalak, and Ashok K. Mahapatra

10. Complex Split Cord Malformations   99
    Shweta Kedia, Ramesh Doddamani, and Ashok K. Mahapatra

11. Prophylactic Surgery in Split Cord Malformations   111
    Vivek Tandon, Skanda Moorthy, and Ashok K. Mahapatra

12. Protocol for Management of Split Cord Malformations   119
    Vivek Tandon, Harish Chandrappa, and Ashok K. Mahapatra

13. Long-Term Outcome of Split Cord Malformations   133
    Manoj Phalak and Ashok K. Mahapatra

14. Anesthesia for Neural Tube Defects   139
    Ashutosh Kaushal and Ashish Bindra

Index   153

Preface

Split cord malformation (SCM) is a rare condition. This condition was earlier named as diastematomyelia and diplomyelia. During my 6 months' pediatric surgery posting in surgical residency way back in 1976, I had never seen a patient with SCM, as it was difficult to diagnose this condition without a CT or MRI. The pediatric surgery unit of All India Institute of Medical Sciences (AIIMS), New Delhi, India, was running a hydrocephalus clinic, and meningomyelocele (MMC) were being operated upon by pediatric surgeons, mostly in cases of emergency, as many patients came with rupture or at an impending rupture stage. No specific investigations were done for babies. To me, at that time, operations were by and large successful. No one knew what the underlying pathology was and what happened to the patients afterwards.

My senior residency (1979–1982) had a good exposure to neurosurgical cases, including ventriculoatrial (VA) and ventriculoperitoneal (VP) shunts for adults, many with hydrocephalus due to tuberculous meningitis (TBM) or tumor-related obstructive hydrocephalus. Exposure to tumor surgery, neurovascular surgery, neurotrauma, and even functional neurosurgery was good at that point in time. Over 1000 patients were operated upon each year for neurosurgical problems. However, pediatric neurosurgery, including surgery for spinal dysraphism (SD), was still rare. I had gone through the *Textbook of Neurosurgery* by Youman and *Pediatric Neurosurgery* by Prof Donald Matson and Prof Ingraham. But knowledge of pediatric neurosurgery in the late 1970s and early 1980s, I must confess, was rudimentary. Hence, for me, starting surgery for neural tube defects (NTD) at AIIMS was challenging, as MRI was also not available at that time; mostly, CT scans were done for such cases.

In 1980, scoliosis surgery started at AIIMS, and Harrington instrumentation was started by the orthopedics department headed by Prof P. K. Dave. During those days, no specific investigations were carried out in patients of idiopathic scoliosis. Two young patients deteriorated after Harrington instrumentation. It was a wake-up call for orthopedicians performing scoliosis surgery. Then, in the mid-1980s, a protocol was developed to carry out MRI in all cases of scoliosis and other deformities. That is how we slowly started recognizing and diagnosing an increasing number of SCMs.

SCM is not a common condition. However, with the workload of pediatric neurosurgery increasing steadily from 1985 to 2000, we started getting over 250 to 300 cases of SD in a year, and roughly 50% to 60% used to get operated as adequate beds were not available. Thus, in a year, around 130 to 160 patients could be operated for SD and they were broadly divided into three groups: (1) one-third pure MMC, (2) one-third lipoma, and (3) one-third SCM, and among them, 10% had combination of SCM with MMC, SCM with MMC and lipoma, or SCM with lipoma. This had given us impetus to work on lipoma, SCM, tethered cord syndrome (TCS), and adult TCS in order to find out how we fare as compared to the rest of the world, with ours being a large referral center with all facilities, and cases from various states with lipoma and SCM used to get referred to me at AIIMS. I was able to build up a large series of cases. Over the years, an increasing number of young faculty joined, and pediatric neurosurgery, by the year 2000, had picked up momentum and people had started talking about SCM, lipoma, neuromonitoring, and more importantly, Pang's theory. I met my dear friend, Prof D. Pang, at a world congress in Morocco in 2005. I was enthralled and shared my experience regarding SCM. Subsequently, a large number of my friends and pediatric neurosurgeons visited AIIMS and saw our pediatric neurosurgical activities and, more importantly, management of SCM and lipoma. Some of my friends who visited AIIMS between 2002 and 2012 were Prof Steinbock, Prof Di Rocco, Prof D. Pang, Prof Oi, Prof Venturia, Prof Solanki, Prof Perry Kahan, Prof Tomita, and many others. We also published many papers on SCM, lipoma, myelocystoceles, and TCS. Thus, AIIMS Neurosurgery could be recognized as a center doing a lot of pediatric neurosurgery, especially NTD.

This book has been long due. SCM is not that uncommon in India, and with our vast experience on this subject, it is appropriate to publish a book and highlight the way an SCM patient must be treated to get excellent results. This book has 14 chapters dealing with all aspects of SCM, including embryology, diagnosis, and management.

Over the years, classification has evolved as we are understanding various aspects of SCM. Classification does guide us for proper management. Simple SCM and complex SCM are different, so also the ventral versus dorsal spur. These things can be diagnosed preoperatively and can be successfully managed.

Management of type II SCMs is simple. However, type Id and dorsal or dorsoventral spur, arising from spinous process and going ventrally, need special care to prevent spinal cord damage. That is why a separate chapter is written on dorsal spur. Complex SCMs are also a challenge. The associated pathology like MMC, lipoma, thick filum, and congenital tumors must be managed on their own merit. Hence, proper diagnosis of the complex SCM helps in planning surgical strategy.

The role of prophylactic surgery and age for undergoing surgery still remain controversial, as many pediatric neurosurgeons do not contemplate surgery in asymptomatic cases. Anesthesia consideration is very important in planning surgery in infants; however, above 5 years, it may not be a problem. It needs training, skill, and experience to deal with infants. Hence, this topic is also covered, so that an understanding of comprehensive management of SCM can be delivered to our students and readers. Thus, I believe this book is going to enrich our students and young faculty who want to pursue pediatric neurosurgery as a future career.

Ashok K. Mahapatra, MS, MCh, DNB, MAMS, FNAS

About the Authors

Ashok K. Mahapatra, MS, MCh, DNB, MAMS, FNAS

Ashok K. Mahapatra is currently the Vice-Chancellor of Siksha 'O' Anusandhan (SOA) University, Bhubaneswar. Prior to joining SOA, he worked at AIIMS, New Delhi, from where he retired in December 2017 as Dean (Research) and Chief of Neurosciences Centre. He was also Head of the Department of Neurosurgery from 2009 to 2012, when he joined as Founding Director at AIIMS, Bhubaneswar, where he started MBBS, 2012; BSc Nursing, 2013; and BSc. Medical Technology, 2014; and a 600-bedded hospital. From 2006 to 2009, he was Director of SGPGI Lucknow. He has written 16 books, published 730 papers in journals, and contributed 145 chapters in edited volumes. He has over 14,000 citations with his H index-55 and 1-10 index 355. He has mentored over 250 neurosurgeons at AIIMS and SGPGI when he worked at those places. He has operated over 2,500 cases of SD, over 400 SCMs, and 300 spinal lipomas. He has published around 35 papers on SCM and lipoma in the last 25 years.

Sachin A. Borkar, MCh, FACS, DNB, MNAMS

Sachin A. Borkar is currently working as Additional Professor of Neurosurgery at AIIMS, New Delhi, India. He has a lot of accolades to his credit in a glorious academic career, including gold medals during MBBS and DNB Neurosurgery. He has published more than 125 articles in peer-reviewed journals along with 10 chapters in books. He is well-experienced in all aspects of pediatric neurosurgery, including SCM.

Subhashree Mahapatra, BSc, MSc, PhD

Subhashree Mahapatra is a scientist who studied BSc (Hons) in human biology at AIIMS, New Delhi, and MSc in Biotechnology at JNU, New Delhi. She completed her PhD in Molecular Medicine from Hannover Medical University, Germany, in 2012. For the last 8 years, she has worked on skin allergy, its molecular aspect, and asthma at various places. She has published 5 papers and 4 chapters. She has helped Professor Ashok K. Mahapatra in editing the manuscripts.

Contributors

Amol Raheja, MCh
Assistant Professor
Department of Neurosurgery
All India Institute of Medical Sciences
New Delhi, India

Ashish Bindra, MD, DM
Additional Professor
Department of Neuroanaesthesia & Critical Care
All India Institute of Medical Sciences
New Delhi, India

Ashok K. Mahapatra, MS, MCh, DNB, MAMS, FNAS
Vice-Chancellor
Siksha 'O' Anusandhan University
Bhubaneshwar, Odisha;
Former Chief of Neurosciences Center
Former Head
Department of Neurosurgery
All India Institute of Medical Sciences
New Delhi, India

Ashutosh Agrawal, MCh
Ex-Senior Resident
Department of Neurosurgery
All India Institute of Medical Sciences
New Delhi, India

Ashutosh Kaushal, MD
Ex-Senior Resident
Department of Neuroanaesthesia & Critical Care
All India Institute of Medical Sciences
New Delhi, India

Dattaraj P. Sawarkar, MS, MCh
Associate Professor
Department of Neurosurgery
All India Institute of Medical Sciences
New Delhi, India

Deepak K. Gupta, MS, MCh, PhD
Professor
Department of Neurosurgery
All India Institute of Medical Sciences
New Delhi, India

Harish Chandrappa, MCh
Ex-Senior Resident
Department of Neurosurgery
All India Institute of Medical Sciences
New Delhi, India

Kanwaljeet Garg, MCh
Associate Professor
Department of Neurosurgery
All India Institute of Medical Sciences
New Delhi, India

Manoj Phalak, MCh
Associate Professor
Department of Neurosurgery
All India Institute of Medical Sciences
New Delhi, India

Mohit Agrawal, MCh
Ex-Senior Resident
Department of Neurosurgery
All India Institute of Medical Sciences
New Delhi, India

Pankaj Kumar Singh, MS, MCh
Additional Professor
Department of Neurosurgery
All India Institute of Medical Sciences
New Delhi, India

Rajesh Meena, MS, MCh
Assistant Professor
Department of Neurosurgery
All India Institute of Medical Sciences
New Delhi, India

Ramesh Doddamani, MS, MCh
Associate Professor
Department of Neurosurgery
All India Institute of Medical Sciences
New Delhi, India

Ravi Sreenivasan, MS
Assistant Professor
Central Institute of Orthopedics
Safdarjung Hospital
New Delhi, India

Sachin A. Borkar, MCh, FACS, DNB, MNAMS
Additional Professor
Department of Neurosurgery
All India Institute of Medical Sciences
New Delhi, India

Sanjeev A. Sreenivasan, MS, MCh
Ex-Senior Resident
Department of Neurosurgery
All India Institute of Medical Sciences
New Delhi, India

Shweta Kedia, MS, MCh
Associate Professor
Department of Neurosurgery
All India Institute of Medical Sciences
New Delhi, India

Skanda Moorthy, MCh
Ex-Senior Resident
Department of Neurosurgery
All India Institute of Medical Sciences
New Delhi, India

Tarang K. Vora, MS, MCh
Pediatric Neurosurgery Fellow
Department of Neurosurgery
All India Institute of Medical Sciences
New Delhi, India

Vivek Tandon, MS, MCh
Additional Professor
Department of Neurosurgery
All India Institute of Medical Sciences
New Delhi, India

CHAPTER 1

Introduction to Split Cord Malformations

Amol Raheja, Sanjeev A. Sreenivasan, and Ashok K. Mahapatra

Table of Contents

- Introduction 3

- Embryogenesis 3

- Clinical Profile... 4

- Diagnostic Imaging and Radiological Workup 4

- Principles of Management.. 4

Introduction to Split Cord Malformations

Amol Raheja, Sanjeev A. Sreenivasan, and Ashok K. Mahapatra

Introduction

Over decades, the nomenclature for patients with double spinal cords have been changed from diplomyelia or diastematomyelia initially to the currently accepted split cord malformations (SCM), due to the implications of their disparate embryogenesis, dubiety in their terminology, and conflicting usage.[1,2] Multiple initial hypotheses for the genesis of SCM included disorder of notochord genesis, germ layer segregation, or neurulation. However, the most widely accepted hypothesis is the Pang's unified theory of embryogenesis, which proposes that a common ontogenetic error leads to double cord malformations vis à vis formation of adhesions between endoderm and ectoderm, ultimately culminating into an endomesenchymal tract surrounding persistent accessory neurenteric canal that bisects the developing notochord into duplicate hemineural plates.[1,2] This modified state of developing hemineural plates and embryogenetic destiny of endomesenchymal tract constituents govern the final configuration of hemicords and nature of midline septum. This hypothesis also explains the high incidence of fore- and midgut anomalies as well as open myelodysplastic and cutaneous lesions associated with SCM.[1,2] The unique morphology of SCM acquired by each patient depends on three embryogenetic fates of the endomesenchymal tract: (1) variable extent to which endomesenchymal tract persists; (2) the embryo's ability to heal around endomesenchymal tract; and (3) the cumulative destiny of dislocated midline mesoderm and endoderm.[1,2]

Pang further subclassified SCM into type I and II, based on median septum characteristics and dural tube status surrounding the two hemicords.[1,2] SCM type II consists of single dural tube housing two hemicords, which are separated by a fibrous median septum that is nonrigid. On the contrary, SCM type I houses each hemicord in its own dural tube, and they are separated by a rigid osseocartilaginous midline septum.[1,2] All other associated tethering elements in SCM such as centromedian vascular structures, myelomeningocele manqué, and paramedian nerve roots do overlap between SCM types I and II; hence, there are no consistent differentiating criteria.[1,2] This currently acceptable classification helps subdivide SCM cases preoperatively, based on the radiological imaging, and further plan their surgical management and risk assessment accordingly.[1,3,4] This chapter has been conceptualized to understand the embryogenesis, clinical presentation, diagnostic imaging, radiological workup, decision-making process, and surgical strategy in management of patients with SCM in a nutshell. A detailed discussion will be conducted separately in further chapters.

Embryogenesis

The key differentiating step between formation of SCM-I and SCM-II is the recruitment of meninx primitiva precursor cells during mesenchymal investment over endomesenchymal tract.[2] Pluripotent cells of endomesenchymal tract could develop into a variety of tissues, including lymphoid tissue, blood vessels, dermoid cysts, tubular epithelia, muscle tissue, ganglion cells, fetal renal tissue and, rarely, teratomas, in addition to osseocartilaginous tissue seen in SCM.[3] Similarly, endodermal remnants may present as neurenteric cyst or intestinal duplication.[2,3] Involvement of surface ectoderm by dorsal endomesenchymal tract may manifest in the form of hypertrichosis, capillary hemangioma, etc.[2,3,5,6]

Clinical Profile

SCM is noticed in approximately 20% of children with neural tube defects.[1,4,6] Neurological deficits are seen in both type I and type II SCMs. They may present with occult clinical findings such as scoliosis, lower limb deformities, or cutaneous markers, which act as surrogate markers for underlying SCM.[1,3,4,6] Majority of SCMs are seen in lumbosacral region, followed by dorsal and cervical region. Tethered cord syndrome symptomatology is also evident in SCM.[1,2,4,5,6,8] Severe dysesthetic pain in legs and perineum, followed by sensory and motor deficits, are the common presentation features in adults. On the contrary, pediatric patients present with gait disturbance, followed by pain and progressive foot or spinal deformities.[1,2,4,5,6,8] Delayed bowel and bladder involvement can also be commonly seen. A constellation of systemic anomalies is commonly associated with patients afflicted with SCM, which may include cardiovascular anomalies, urogenital anomalies, and anorectal malformations.[7]

Diagnostic Imaging and Radiological Workup

Over decades, diagnostic imaging of choice for evaluation and planning management of SCM has changed from CT myelogram in the past to MRI in the present era.[1,3,4,6] High likelihood of progressive and irreversible neurological deterioration in unrecognized SCM cases justifies radiological screening of every child with surrogate markers of spinal dysraphism.[1,3] Routine protocol of radiological workup for children with suspected spinal dysraphism should include a panel of noncontrast MRI of the suspected site and screening of the whole brain and spine to exclude any associated hydrocephalus, Chiari malformation, or multisite spinal dysraphism.[1,3,4,6] Ultrasonography of abdomen, renal scans, and urodynamic studies are part of additional systemic workup for these patients, as it can find associated congenital anomalies.[1,3,4,6]

Principles of Management

In general, if a SCM is identified, it should be surgically managed, because its detrimental effect on the spinal cord is unrelated to the state of neural placode under consideration.[1,3] Early intervention to release tethering elements is the treatment of choice for symptomatic patients with SCM and asymptomatic patients with SCM type I.[1,4] On the contrary, there is less convincing evidence in the current literature for asymptomatic tethered cord patients with type II SCM, especially in adult patients.[1,8] Risk of precipitation of neurological deterioration following trauma in adults with physically active lifestyle justifies operating upon such patients, even though asymptomatic.[1,3,8] However, older asymptomatic adults leading sedentary lifestyles can probably be subjected to conservative management. In general, pain responds best to surgical detethering and still remains the best indication for surgery, especially among adult patients with SCM.[1,3,8,9] Sensorimotor deficits, on the other hand, are the next best responder; however, only new onset deficits tend to improve. Finally, bowel-bladder involvement improves only in approximately 40% of patients, although another fraction of patients may have stabilization of their previously progressive bladder/bowel symptoms.[1,3,8] On the contrary, progressive foot deformity may still ensue after adequate detethering of the cord, which is believed to be due to irreversible osseoligamentous changes, which are no longer affected by the existing neurological status. All the tethering lesions should be operated upon in the same surgical session, preferably in a top-down approach, in order to prevent inadvertent and undue stretching of spinal cord after releasing lower tethering elements.[1,3,4,6,8,9]

References

1. Pang D. Split cord malformation: part II—clinical syndrome. Neurosurgery 1992;31(3):481–500
2. Pang D, Dias MS, Ahab-Barmada M. Split cord malformation: part I—a unified theory of embryogenesis for double spinal cord malformations. Neurosurgery 1992;31(3):451–480
3. Erşahin Y. Split cord malformation types I and II: a personal series of 131 patients. Childs Nerv Syst 2013;29(9):1515–1526
4. Mahapatra AK. Split cord malformation: a study of 300 cases at AIIMS 1990–2006. J Pediatr Neurosci 2011;6(Suppl 1):S41–S45
5. Jindal A, Mahapatra AK. Split cord malformations: a clinical study of 48 cases. Indian Pediatr 2000;37(6):603–607
6. Mahapatra AK, Gupta DK. Split cord malformations: a clinical study of 254 patients and a proposal for a new clinical-imaging classification. J Neurosurg 2005;103(6, Suppl):531–536
7. Ozturk E, Sonmez G, Mutlu H, et al. Split-cord malformation and accompanying anomalies. J Neuroradiol 2008;35(3):150–156
8. Pang D, Wilberger JE Jr. Tethered cord syndrome in adults. J Neurosurg 1982;57(1):32–47
9. Sinha S, Agarwal D, Mahapatra AK. Split cord malformations: an experience of 203 cases. Childs Nerv Syst 2006;22(1):3–7

CHAPTER 2

Embryology of Split Cord Malformations

Ashutosh Agarwal, Shweta Kedia, and Ashok K. Mahapatra

Table of Contents

- Introduction 9

- Normal Early Human Embryo Development
  (Journey from 2-Layered to 3-Layered Structure)...... 9

- Embryogenesis of Human NTDs 12

Embryology of Split Cord Malformations

Ashutosh Agarwal, Shweta Kedia, and Ashok K. Mahapatra

Introduction

Split cord malformation (SCM) defines the group of disorders where the spinal cord is split into two by either a bony or fibrous septum. Based on the nature of the dividing structure, it has been classified into types I and II. However, there have been several reports in the literature where complex multilevel splits are described—some of them in association with other congenital disorders. The pathogenesis of complex SCM has always been intriguing and there is still an ongoing search for the explanation of these presentations based on embryology. Authors intend to go through the natural embryological process in this chapter and also analyze the proposed theories of embryogenesis as described in literature.

Normal Early Human Embryo Development (Journey from 2-Layered to 3-Layered Structure)

■ Gastrulation

In the postovulatory days (POD) 1 to 13, which is the first 2 weeks postfertilization, the human embryo cells divide and undergo rearrangements. It results in the formation of a blastocyst, a two-layered embryo suspended between the amniotic and yolk sacs. This is followed by formation of epiblasts on the dorsal surface of embryo and hypoblast on the ventral surface by postovulatory day 4. Prochordal plate is formed by the thickening of the cranial end of the embryo by postovulatory day 13.

This is also the time when primitive streak develops at the caudal end of the embryo and progresses cranially over the next 3 days. By day 16, it has obtained its full length. It is in the midline in the caudal half. The regression of the primitive streak begins thereafter, and it moves back toward the caudal pole of the embryo. Meanwhile, epiblasts migrate toward the primitive streak through the primitive groove running along the length of the primitive streak. Future endodermal cells ingress and displace the ventrally placed hypoblast cells laterally and form the endoderm. With the regression of the streak, future mesodermal cells ingress between the epiblast and endoderm to form the definitive mesoderm. The epiblast cells that are remaining now spread out and replace the ingressed cells to form both the neuroectoderm and surface ectoderm. It should thus be remembered that the embryonic endo-, meso-, and ectoderm are all derivatives of the epiblast.

The Hensen node needs special mention. Located at the cranial end of the primitive streak, this node acts as the organizer of the embryo. It is through this node that the future endodermal cells migrate, as the streak is elongating, and the future notochordal cells are laid down in the midline between the neuroectoderm and endoderm as the notochordal process.

Prospective neuroectoderm have been localized on the epiblast area surrounding the Hensen node toward the rostral half of the primitive streak. Neuroepithelium can be divided into areas that contribute to multiple neuraxial levels.

■ Timeline

- POD 4: Formation of epiblast and hypoblast.
- POD 13: Prochordal plate formed at the cranial end.
- POD 16: Primitive streak obtains full length at caudal end.
- POD 23-25: True notochord is formed.
- POD 24-25: Cranial neuropore closes.
- POD 25-27: Caudal neuropore closes.

■ Notochord Formation

This process starts postovulatory day 16 onward. Cord of cells arranged radially around the notochordal canal constitutes notochordal process. This notochordal canal is in continuity with the amniotic cavity dorsally through the primitive pit. It is between postovulatory days 17 and 21 that the notochordal process elongates. Fusion with the underlying endoderm happens between postovulatory days 18 to 20 and results in the formation of notochordal plate. The notochordal plate gets incorporated into the yolk sac roof and establishes the continuity of notochordal canal. On postovulatory days 17 to 19, neurenteric canal is formed (**Fig. 2.1**). The "true notochord" is formed by postovulatory days 23 to 25, when the plate folds dorsoventrally and separates from the endoderm. This results in obliteration of the neurenteric canal, and continuity with the amniotic and yolk sacs is closed.

Formation of the Neural Tube

By postovulatory day 16, the neuroectoderm is present in the form of pseudostratified columnar epithelium. This overlies the midline notochord and continues laterally, transitioning into squamous epithelium of the cutaneous ectoderm. Neural groove is now visible as a shallow midline fold above the midline notochord on postovulatory days 17 to 19. This groove deepens and forms the neural folds laterally by postovulatory days 19 to 21. These neural folds then elevate and converge toward the midline. They meet to form a closed neural tube. The cutaneous ectoderm apposes and fuses first, followed by neuroectoderm. The disjunction involving the separation of neuroectoderm from cutaneous ectoderm then follows.

Neural tube closure happens over a 4- to 6-day period. Caudal rhombencephalon or cranial spinal cord closes first. Now, it is accepted that this closure happens in several waveforms along the craniocaudal axis rather than in a linear manner like a zipper. The cranial neuropore closes on postovulatory days 24 to 25 in a coordinated fashion with at least four waves interacting. On postovulatory days 25 to 27, caudal neuropore closes. By this time, there are nearly 25 somites formed. Just below the last visible somite, the caudal neuropore is located. The site of closure can be assessed by calculating the distance between the last visible somite and the caudal neuropore. By this calculation, it can be assumed that the

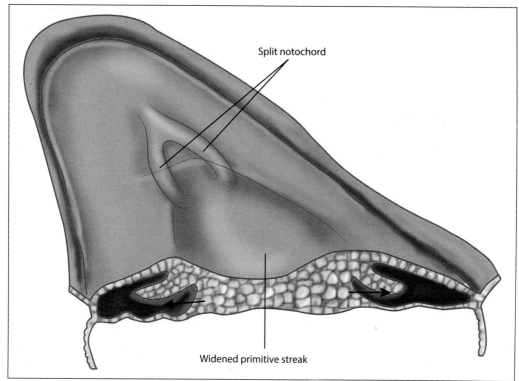

Fig. 2.1 View from above onto the dorsal surface. The caudal pole of the embryo is oriented toward 11 o'clock. During gastrulation, if the primitive streak is abnormally wide, prospective notochordal cells in Hensen's node may begin ingressing more laterally than usual. The paired notochordal streams would not integrate into a single midline notochord and would remain instead as paired paramedian notochordal processes. The caudal neuroepithelium induced by the paired notochordal processes would fail to integrate into a single midline neural plate and would form paired "hemineural plates" instead. Totipotent tissue from Hensen's node could pass into the gap between the two notochordal processes and form a number of different caudal tissue types.

spinal cord almost as far as S2 is formed by primary neurulation, and secondary neurulation involves formation of the terminal filum and maybe the lower sacral spinal cord.

Secondary Neurulation

After the caudal neuropore has closed on postovulatory days 25 to 27, the entire nervous system is covered with skin and more caudal neural development occurs by secondary neurulation. By this time, primitive streak remnants have regressed to form a caudal cell mass (CCM) at the caudal embryonic pole. This CCM extends from the posterior neuropore to the cloacal membrane and composed of multipotent cells.

The mechanism described for secondary neurulation is specific to each species. Human secondary neurulation closely resembles that of the mouse. As per Müller and O'Rahilly, neural cord here is in continuity with the primary neural tube. It has a single lumen, which is continuous with the central canal of the primary neural tube.

Lemire and Bolli believe there is a resemblance to the neurulation process of chick embryos. They described multiple independent secondary tubes with separate lumina and no identifiable connections with one another or the primary neural tube.

Occlusion of the Spinal Neurocele

Between postovulatory days 23 to 32 while the neural tube is closing and also after it, there is temporary occlusion of the central lumen, because of the apposition of the lateral walls of the neural tube. This occlusion starts cranially beyond the first pair of somites and goes as far caudally as the ninth somite involving 60% of the neuraxis. The neural tube located cranially beyond occlusion expands rapidly because of its growth and expansion of the ventricular system. The closed cranial neuropore and the occluded caudal neural tube helps in isolating the cranial ventricular system. This isolated ventricular system has an intraluminal pressure, providing a driving force for brain growth. One of the mechanisms responsible for Chiari malformation is the failure to maintain this driving force in patients with open neural tube.

Embryogenesis of Human NTDs

Von Recklinghausen proposed the nonclosure of neural tube theory for explaining the neural tube defects.

Pang et al proposed a unified theory on the embryogenesis of SCM and suggested the error occurs almost at the same time as the primitive neurenteric canal is closing. The "accessory neurenteric canal" is formed through the midline embryonic disc. This establishes the communication between yolk sac and amnion and is the basis of error. This accessory neurenteric canal allows continued contact between ectoderm and endoderm and results in regional "splitting" of the notochord and the overlying neural plate. Elsewhere, it is rolled up to form the neural tube. The site of the fistula is variable but always cranial to the primitive neurenteric canal and explains why all SCMs involve cord segments that are rostral to the coccyx. The normal neurenteric canal opens into the primitive pit, which lies opposite the coccyx. Endomesenchymal tract is formed by the condensation of mesenchyme around this abnormal fistula. This occupies the space between the split notochord and split neural plate and may contain precursor cells from the meninx primitiva. In the presence of meninx primitiva cells, there is the formation of a bony septum, resulting in type I SCM. In the absence of it, a fibrous band would result in the formation of type II SCM. The composite type of SCMs may form when there are multiple accessory canals (**Fig. 2.2**).

Generally, in SCM type I, a single bony spur arises from the posterior surface of the vertebral body. However, there may be occasions when the spur arises from the posterior arch. Chandra et al proposed two hypotheses for posterior origin of bony spur including: (1) ventral cell mass gets disconnected after dorsal migration of meninx primitiva cells and (2) the other possibility being initial migration of meninx primitiva cells around the hemicords instead of between them to accumulate along the dorsal arch.

Others like Dias et al have recently proposed that problems in the midline axial integration during gastrulation may also be responsible for several myelomeningoceles. The Hensen node fails to lay down a single notochord. The authors suggest that during gastrulation each half of the Hensen node gives rise to paired notochordal analgen. On either side of the node, two independent hemineural plates grow

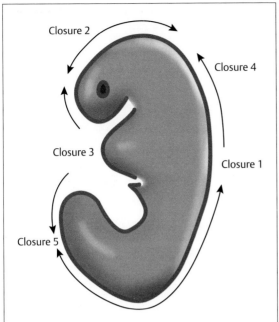

Fig. 2.2 Modified human concept based on mouse multisite closure, as used for retrospective interpretation of human neural tube defects (NTDs).

and subsequently develop into a hemicord. If neurulation fails in one hemicord, hemimyelomenigocele happens. If it fails in both the hemicords, it results in myelomeningocele associated with an SCM (**Fig. 2.3**). Multipotent cells contained within the Hensen node are responsible for the varied associated malformations like neurenteric cysts, combined spina bifida (split notochord syndrome), and other entities between the two hemicords.

Enough evidence supports genetic cause for neural tube defects (NTDs). The fact that the first-degree relatives of patients are at a high risk of NTDs is a pointer toward genetic involvement. The risk of the sibling having NTD is 2 to 3%, and with the third child, the risk increases to 10%. The incidence of NTDs is varied for different populations. Concordance rates vary between 3.7 and 18% in monozygotic twin pairs. NTDs may also be seen in association with known genetic and chromosomal anomalies (such as Waardenberg syndrome, Trisomy 13 and 18).

Variety of molecular involvements have been shown in NTDs including transcription factors and coactivators, signal transducers, folate binding proteins, tumor suppressor gene products, cytoskeletal components, DNA methyltransferases, nuclear and cell membrane receptors, chromosomal proteins, gap junction proteins, cell surface receptors, and actin regulators and binding proteins. These may be related to specific types of NTDs. Each may involve disruption of specific waves of neural tube closure and can be disrupted without interfering with other waves. Genes controlling folate metabolism and methyltransferase reactions involving methionine and homocysteine have caught recent attention. Supplementing periconceptional folate to pregnant women have shown reduction in the incidence of NTDs both in women known to have child with NTDs and without.

Almost half of NTDs may be caused by factors that are independent of folate mechanisms. Teratogens too may be contributing to various cellular mechanisms causing NTDs in humans. Valproic acid is known

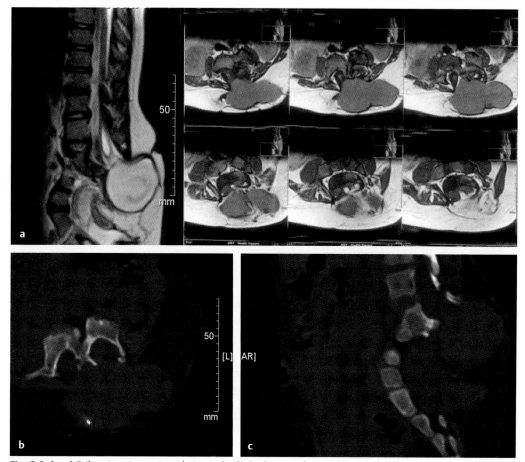

Fig. 2.3 (a–c) Failure in primary neurulation in both the hemicords results in myelomenigocoele associated with SCM type I.

to cause NTDs in humans. The most likely mechanism of teratogenic effect being inhibition of neural fold fusion, as the folate metabolic pathways is disrupted because of interference in conversion of tetrahydrofolate to 5-formyltetrahydro-folate.

Suggested Readings

Borkar SA, Mahapatra AK. Split cord malformations: a two years experience at AIIMS. Asian J Neurosurg 2012;7(2):56–60

Chandra PS, Kamal R, Mahapatra AK. An unusual case of dorsally situated bony spur in a lumbar split cord malformation. Pediatr Neurosurg 1999;31(1):49–52

Dias MS, Partington M. Embryology of myelomeningocele and anencephaly. Neurosurg Focus 2004;16(2):E1

Mahapatra AK, Gupta DK. Split cord malformations: a clinical study of 254 patients and a proposal for a new clinical-imaging classification. J Neurosurg 2005;103(6, Suppl):531–536

Pang D, Dias MS, Ahab-Barmada M. Split cord malformation: part I—a unified theory of embryogenesis for double spinal cord malformations. Neurosurgery 1992;31(3):451–480

Classification of Split Cord Malformations

Dattaraj P. Sawarkar, Deepak K. Gupta, and Ashok K. Mahapatra

Table of Contents

■ Introduction 17

■ Pang's Classification 17

■ Composite Split Cord Malformations 19

■ Location of Spur 20

■ Completeness of Spur 21

■ Number of Spurs 21

■ SCMs Associated with Other Spinal/Cranial
  Dysraphisms 21

■ Spur with Intracranial or Extracranial
  Malformations 23

■ New Proposal for Type I Split Cord Malformation
  by Mahapatra and Gupta 23

■ Embryological Basis of SCMs 24

■ Clinical Features 25

■ Diagnosis 26

■ Treatment and Outcome 26

■ Conclusions 27

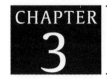

CHAPTER 3

Classification of Split Cord Malformations

Dattaraj P. Sawarkar, Deepak K. Gupta, and Ashok K. Mahapatra

Introduction

Occult spinal dysraphism[1] is not an uncommon clinical entity in neurosurgical practice. Split cord malformation (SCM) is a rare form of spinal dyraphism characterized by a split along the midline of the cord, dividing it into two symmetric or asymmetric entities housed in same or separate dural tubes. SCMs represent up to 5% of the outpatient pediatric population with congenital spinal anomalies. Most of the patients are children and they present to their physician in infancy or early childhood. Age groups commonly presenting with these disorders are 4 to 7 years and 12 to 15 years;[2] the latter being a result of the growth spurt around puberty, which unmasks certain clinical features. Presence of neurocutaneous markers is a hallmark sign on first clinical examination. SCMs are congenital disorders where there is division of the spinal cord into two halves by a bony or fibrous spur. Cohen and Sledge[3] described diastematomyelia as a cleft or split within the spinal cord. Diplomyelia, coined by von Recklinghausen, is the presence of a separate cord-like structure dorsal or ventral to the original cord. Dimyelia is the presence of two true separated spinal cords within two distinct dural sacs. However, many of these terms were utilized interchangeably in the literature.

Over the years, various classifications have been described in the literature for SCMs.

Pang's Classification

The unified theory of embryogenesis was first described by Pang et al,[4,5] classifying the SCMs in two types:

1. Type I SCM: It comprises two dural sacs separated in the midline by a bony spur. There is fusion of the lamina to the adjacent levels, and these laminae are often hypertrophic. CT scan examination reveals a bony spur. Type I SCM is usually characterized by presence of spina bifida defect and fusion of adjacent segments. These are most commonly located in the lumbar region (**Fig. 3.1** and **Fig. 3.2**).

2. Type II SCM: It comprises a single dural sac encasing two hemicords. These are tethered to the dura via a fibrous band. MRI reveals two separate hemicords within a single subarachnoid space. Presence of fibrous strand can be demonstrated on a high-resolution MR. This may be located anywhere along the neuraxis.

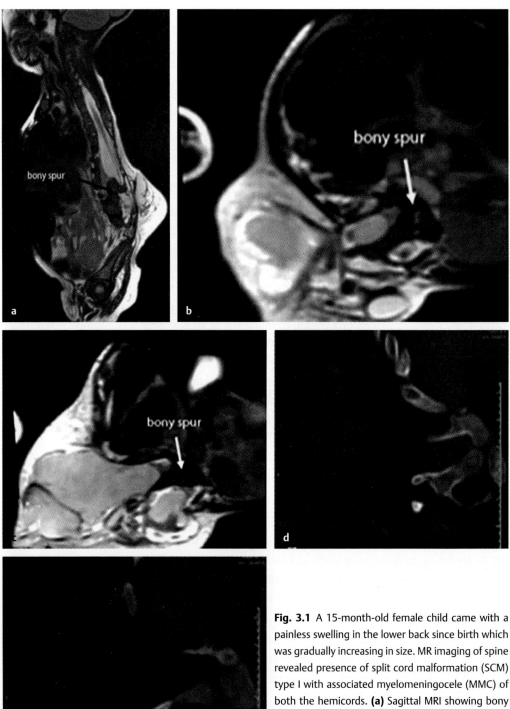

Fig. 3.1 A 15-month-old female child came with a painless swelling in the lower back since birth which was gradually increasing in size. MR imaging of spine revealed presence of split cord malformation (SCM) type I with associated myelomeningocele (MMC) of both the hemicords. **(a)** Sagittal MRI showing bony spur. **(b)** Axial MRI image showing type I SCM and image **(c)** showing bony spur with MMC of both hemicords. **(d, e)** Images showing CT scan axial cuts showing bony spur.

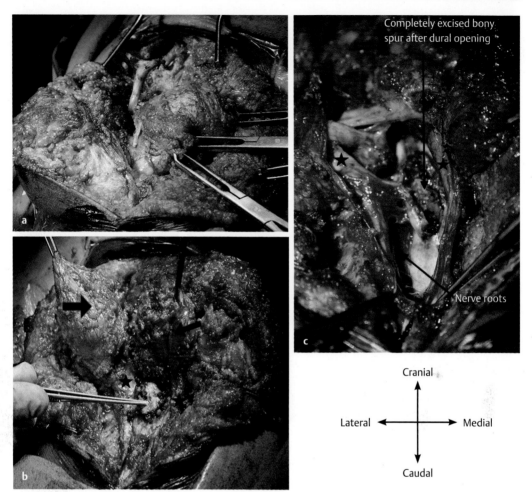

Fig. 3.2 Intraoperative pictures of Fig. 3.1 patient. **(a)** Image showing bony spur. **(b)** Intraoperative image after excision of bony spur showing two separate dural tubes. **(c)** Intraoperative image showing two hemispinal cords after dural opening. (Reprinted with permission from Meena RK, Doddamani RS, Sharma R. Contiguous diastematomyelia with lipomyelomeningocele in each hemicord—an exceptional case of spinal dysraphism. World Neurosurg. 2019 Mar;123:103–107.)

Composite Split Cord Malformations

Some patients may have same or both types of SCMs at different levels with normal cord in between. This form of complex dysraphism is called composite SCM. Type I SCM has two hemicords housed in separate dural sheaths with an intervening bony spur, and type II SCM has two hemicords housed in a single dural tube with an intervening fibrous median septum (**Fig. 3.3**). The embryogenesis of such composite SCMs can be explained by the multiple neurenteric canal theory. There can be multiple separate foci of ectoendodermal adhesions and endomesenchymal tracts during the embryogenesis, leading to the development of composite SCMs with an intervening normal cord. This unique presentation of composite

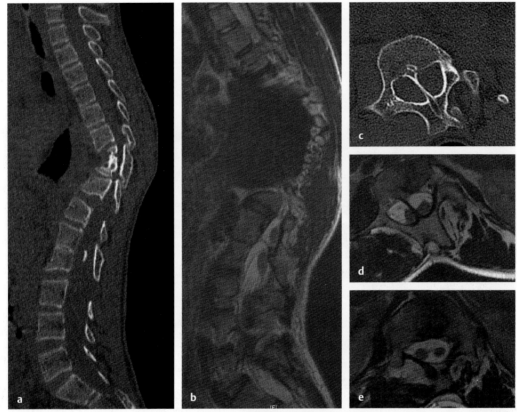

Fig. 3.3 Figure showing composite split cord malformations (SCMs) where both type I and II SCMs are present. Image showing **(a)** sagittal CT and **(b)** sagittal MRI with bony spur at L1 level. **(c)** Axial CT image with the bony spur. **(d)** Axial MRI with a complete bony spur causing splitting of the cord into two hemicords. **(e)** Axial MRI of the same patient with type II split cord malformation at D10 level with normal spinal cord between the two SCMs.

SCMs was noted by Ailawadhi and Mahapatra[6] in a patient having three posterior bony spurs and one fibrous spur at different levels. Similarly, Singh et al[7] reported a patient with long-segment type I SCM and type II SCM at the lower levels. The frequency of composite type SCM has been reported to be less than 1% by Harwood–Nash and McHugh.[8]

Location of Spur

SCMs can also be categorized according to location of spur. It can either be:

- Ventral spur: Proceeding from vertebral body backwards.
- Dorsal spur: Proceeding from lamina towards the vertebral body.

Chandra et al[9] pointed out the presence of dorsally situated spur in 1999.

Completeness of Spur

Classification depending upon completeness of spur:
- Complete spur.
- Incomplete spur.

Number of Spurs

Classification depending upon numbers of spur:
- Single spur.
- Multiple spur.
- Multisegmented spur.

Anatomical-pathological modifications to Pang's classification for type III SCMs were described by Alzhrani et al.[10] They subdivided type III multilevel SCMs into the following: type IIIA: Bony spur at multiple levels, type IIIB: Fibrous septum at multiple levels, and type IIIC: Mixed fibrous and bony spur at multiple levels or with associated anomalies.

SCMs Associated with Other Spinal/Cranial Dysraphisms

- Spur alone.
- Spur with spinal dysraphisms like myelomenigocele (MMC)/myelocystocele/syringomyelia/lipoma/dermoid.
- Spur with cranial malformations like hydrocephalus (HCP)/Chiari/craniosynostosis (**Fig. 3.4**).

Spinal dysraphisms are congenital malformations affecting the spinal cord and vertebral bodies heterogeneously. These malformations can be simple or complex. Contiguous, solitary malformations are termed simple, whereas multiple malformations occurring in combination or in a noncontiguous manner with other organ anomalies are termed complex.

Open form of spinal dysraphisms can present incongruously with SCMs. MMCs have been reported in up to 41% of all SCMs.[11] Clearly, both open and closed forms of spinal dysraphisms can occur together. MMC was reported in 17.4% of SCM patients by Ozturk et al.[12] In their series of 33 patients with MMC, Higashida et al[13] noted three patients (9%) with SCM.

Chiari malformation, HCP, and syrinx are other frequent associations in patients with SCM and MMC,[11,12] complicating the management of these disorders. Usually patients with SCM do not show association with Chiari malformation, but in patients with both SCM and MMC, it is a common occurrence.[13] HCP and syrinx also have been noted to be more common in patients with SCM associated with MMC than in those with pure SCM.[14,15] Myeloschisis associated with SCM has also been reported by Akiyama et al[16] and Yamanaka et al.[17] A case of lumbar SCM with lateral hemimyelomeningocele and associated Chiari II malformation was noted by Rowley and Johnson.[18]

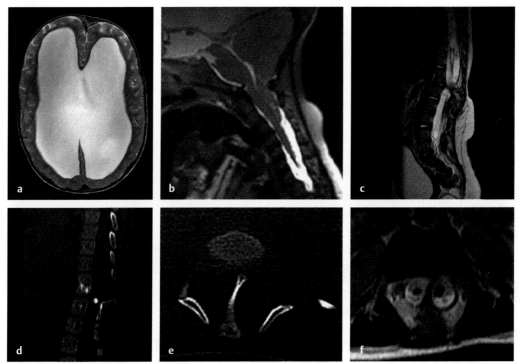

Fig. 3.4 **(a)** A 5-year-old female child with congenital hydrocephalus, **(b)** Chiari II malformation, **(c, d)** sagittal MRI and CT images revealing type I SCM at D12–L1 level, **(e, f)** axial CT and MRI images at that level.

Myelocystocele can also present with SCM. A 4-month-old girl with diastematomyelia, terminal myelocystocele arising from one hemicord, ectopic right kidney, Chiari I malformation, and partial sacral agenesis was reported by Parmar et al.[19] A complex spinal dysraphism with two different level SCMs along with nonterminal myelocystocele, bifid fatty filum, coccygeal dermal sinus, and HCP was reported by Khandelwal et al.[20] A series of 17 and 8 cases of myelocystoceles were noted by Gupta and Mahapatra[21] and Jaiswal and Mahapatra,[22] respectively. Other organ abnormalities such as OEIS complex which include omphalocele (O), exstrophy of bladder (E), imperforate anus (I), and spinal abnormalities (S) are a common occurrence in patients with myelocystocele.[23]

A case of HCP, Chiari malformation, syringohydromyelia, SCM, dermal sinus tract, lumbosacral myelomeningocele, and tethered cord was noted by Emmez et al.[24] A 5-year-old boy with tethered cord, diastometamyelia, spinal dysraphism, terminal lipoma, spinal epidermoid, and dermal sinus tract was reported by Avcu et al.[25] Similarly, a child with a type I SCM associated with hemivertebrae, lipomyelomeningoceles in each hemicord of the SCM, a terminal myelocystocele, and concurrent segmental meningocele was reported by Solanki et al.[26] Two cases of SCM with intraspinal teratoma were reported by Maiti et al,[27] of which one was extradural within meningocele and other intramedullary.

Spur with Intracranial or Extracranial Malformations

- Spur with extracranial malformations (like dextrocadia/renal/gastrointestinal tract [GIT]/lung).
- Spur with intracranial malformations.

Other organ system malformations like genitourinary, cardiac, renal, etc. are frequently associated with spinal dyraphisms. Cases of multiple spinal dysraphic states with situs inversus or dextrocardia have been reported by Dwarakanath et al[28] and Tubbs et al.[29] A complex form of SCMs associated with teratoma, extending into the mediastinum, was noted by Naik et al.[30] A 1-day-old male neonate with multiple right-sided anomalies, hypoplastic right face, decreased movement of the right upper limb with absent right cervical hemivertebrae, right cervical lipomyelomeningocele, and cervical diplomyelia with right hemicord terminating in a blind pouch was reported by Shieh and Lam.[31] Sacral hypoplasia and agenesis of right kidney was reported by Higashida et al[13] in one of their patients with MMC along with SCM.

A classification system should be relevant in terms of its embryology and clinical finding as well as help in planning management, deciding type of surgery, and helping in deciding long-term outcome.

New Proposal for Type I Split Cord Malformation by Mahapatra and Gupta[32,33]

Pang's unified theory of embryogenesis is well-accepted.[4] The theory states all SCMs to be a result of an error in the formation of the accessory neurenteric canal connecting the amnion and the yolk sac. This tract is invested with mesenchyme to form an endomesenchymal tract, splitting the neural plate and the notochord. All types of SCMs cannot be explained by this hypothesis.

To address this shortcoming, a new classification, based on intraoperative findings of spur level and its relation to cord, was put forth by Mahapatra and Gupta.[32,33] Their proposed subclassification of SCM type I is detailed below (**Fig. 3.5**):

1. **Type Ia:** Bony spur in the center, with equally duplicated cord above and below the spur (**Fig. 3.5a**).

2. **Type Ib:** Bony spur at the superior pole with no space above, and a large duplicated cord lower down (**Fig. 3.5b**).

3. **Type Ic:** Bony spur at the lower pole, with a large duplicated cord above (**Fig. 3.5c**).

4. **Type Id:** Bony spur straddling the bifurcation, with no space above or below the spur (**Fig. 3.5d**).

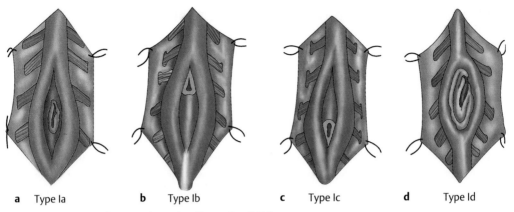

a   Type Ia   b   Type Ib   c   Type Ic   d   Type Id

Fig. 3.5 (a–d) Types of type I split cord malformation (SCM).

SCM type Ia was noted in 48% of cases (12/25) by Mahapatra and Gupta. Postoperative outcome was uneventful in these patients. SCM type Ib was noted in 16% (4/25). Here, the bony spur was seen at the upper level of the split, with two widely separated hemicords below, warranting dissection and removal of the spur from below the split. In SCM type Ic, seen in 12% (3/25), bony spur was noted at the lowermost aspect of the split, with two widely separated hemicords above, warranting dissection and removal of the spur from above the split, as there is a narrow space below. Bony spur found tightly straddling the bifurcation, with no space either above or below the split in SCM type Id. This, being the second most common type, was noted in 6/25 patients (24%). This subtype carried the highest risk of iatrogenic injury to the hemicords. Postoperative neurological deterioration was seen in 67% (4/6) patients with this subtype. It can be concluded that SCM type Ia may be more easy to operate upon and carries lower risk of deterioration in comparison to SCM type Id, where the surgery may require more precision and be more complex due to paucity of space.

Embryological Basis of SCMs

SCMs typically result during the 3rd week of embryological development. In the 1940s, Herren et al described SCM to be a result of excessive infolding of the neural plate.[4] Gardner proposed rupture of the neural tube secondary to hydromyelia as cause for formation of two hemicords. Penetration of mesodermal fibrous tissue into the space between the ruptured neural tubes led to the formation of fibrous or bony spur. Bremer, in his accessory neurenteric canal theory, proposed that the notochord and neural plate is divided into two parts by a diverticulum arising from archenteron, the precursor of the gut.

The patterning of the vertebral system into dorsal and ventral portions is controlled by genes of the *wnt* family. Lack of protocadherin expression in the chick embryos have been noted to cause failed integration of the normally elongated notochordal masses. These present as the regions of split in the cord. An open dorsal diverticulum would subsequently form a dorsal enteric fistula. In the event of disappearance of the endodermal components, all that remains is a fibrous or bony spur separating the two hemicords.

Pang[4] postulated a Unified theory of embryogenesis, according to which an endomesenchymal tract composed of meninx primitiva and bone precursor cells gave origin to SCM type I, that is, a bony septum and associated vertebral malformation. This meninx primitiva typically arises around the 30th day of embryogenesis. Type II SCM forms in the absence of meninx primitiva and bone precursor cells. Theory also stated that caudal midline integration failures coincide with development of meninx primitiva; hence, type I split mostly occurs from L2 to L4. Due to the concurrent development of the neural axis and vertebral elements, intraspinal anomalies, including SCM, can be associated with other congenital spinal deformities. The two main congenital spinal deformities frequently described are congenital scoliosis and kyphosis.

Clinical Features

Spinal cord dysraphism can present in varied forms.[4,34] These children may be asymptomatic till early adulthood. Lumbar spine is the most common location for these lesions. Thoracic and cervical are not common locations for diastematomyelia. Back pain, reduced strength in lower limbs, paraplegia, urinary or bowel incontinence, sensory loss in the lower limbs, persistent nonhealing ulcers in the feet, and equinus/varus deformity of feet may be some of the presenting symptoms. Back pain with radiculopathy can be seen in about 10% patients.

Skin stigmata were frequently reported in approximately half or more than half of patients with SCM, of which hypertrichosis was the most common hallmark. Neurocutaneous markers include dermal sinus, tuft of hair, nevi or hyperpigmented patches on skin, especially in the lower back. Associated spinal deformity[35] like kyphoscoliosis, absent disc at the level of split, and hypertrophic bone where the median spike attaches have also been reported (**Table 3.1**). Congenital scoliosis and MMC are other congenital anomalies which may manifest with SCM (5% and 15%, respectively). Scoliosis is more common in type I SCM and is frequently located at or one level rostral the MMC defect, tethering contributes to progression of scoliosis in these patients.

Due to the rostral migration of the neural elements, with respect to the bony spinal canal, cutaneous markers are commonly located below the level of neural defect.

Table 3.1 Associated anomalies with SCMs[3,36]

Anomaly	Probability of association
Tethered cord/low lying cord	>50%
Kyphoscoliosis	40–60%
Syringomyelia	25–40%
Thickened/fatty filum	
Dermoid cyst	
Dermal sinus/tract	10–25%
Neurenteric cyst	
Spinal lipoma	

Abbreviation: SCMs, split cord malformations.

Nearly 66% patients present with sensory or motor deficits.[5] Morphological asymmetry of the lower limbs is also as common. The commonly seen triad of neuro-orthopedic syndrome consists of limb length discrepancy, muscular atrophy, and foot deformity. However, patients with symmetrical lower limbs may manifest with asymmetric neurological deficit, and this has been related to the underlying hydromyelia within the particular hemicord.

Urodynamic studies are usually indicated in these patients for documentation of urological abnormalities and status of bladder capacity and residual volume.

Diagnosis

Antenatal diagnostic testing includes a second trimester anomaly scan, which can highlight hyperechogenic foci within the spinal canal. Establishing a firm diagnosis needs an MRI of the area of interest, with screening of whole spine and evaluation of ventricle size of brain and presence of associated Chiari malformation or syringomyelia. T1-weighted sequences are usually best indicators of hemicords. Presence of fatty filum, lipoma, or dermal sinus tract can also be appreciated in these images. As much as 90% patients have a low-lying conus medullaris. Presence of two separate dural sleeves and subarachnoid spaces (*owl sign*) can be well made out in T2-weighted images in type I SCM. For studying the bony anatomy of the spur, a CT scan may often suffice. Most commonly, these spurs are noted to rise from the midline of the dorsal aspect of the vertebral body, or obliquely into the spinal canal. Other bony abnormalities which can be identified include bifid vertebrae, hemivertebrae, or butterfly vertebrae. Intersegmental fusion of lamina and presence of bony spina bifida are other features that are specific for type I SCM.

Treatment and Outcome

Progressive symptoms in these patients are attributed to the tethering of the cord, whereas fixed deficits are attributed to malformed nervous tissue during embryogenesis. Detethering as treatment may suffice in most patients, but in type I split, in addition to detethering, the bony spur with medial dural cuff must be removed to reconstitute a single dural tube. Type II SCMs are not known to have any bony spinal abnormality at the level of the split; however, there may be a spina bifida occulta or fatty filum in the lumbosacral region. Here, the cord needs to be detethered at the level of the split and at the level of spina bifida or fatty filum too.

Asymptomatic type II SCM patients, as indicated by previous literature, are also at a risk of neurological deterioration. Hence, prophylactic surgical exploration may be warranted.

Neuromonitoring has an important role to play in surgical management. Use of motor-evoked potentials and sphincter monitoring provides intraoperative assistance. Use of marker X-ray or intraoperative imaging with image intensifier helps in identifying the level of split and associated bony anomaly clearly.

For type I SCM, laminectomy may be needed at the adjacent level to expose the region of interest. Bilateral laminectomies at the level of bony spur is then performed and the two dural sacs are gently isolated by subperiosteal dissection at the spur. The caudal portion of the sac is usually most adherent to the spur. After complete separation from the dural sacs, the spur is gradually resected with a high-speed drill. This is a common step where significant bleeding may be encountered. Then, a midline incision is given to open the dura. The hemicords are dissected away from the dural attachments. Arachnoid adhesions are usually noted to be more dense caudally. Some nonfunctional nerve roots may even cross the dura. A single dural sac is reconstituted after resecting the bands.

Detethering may also treat the syringomyelia indirectly. Postoperatively, patients are nursed in prone position for 24 to 48 hours. Patient is usually mobilized within 48 to 72 hours. Urinary retention (20–25%) is not uncommon in postoperative period, and this usually needs transient catheterization. Cerebrospinal fluid (CSF) leak (5%) and wound infection (3%) are some rare complications and new onset sensory or motor deficits may also be seen infrequently (7%).

Conclusions

Patient with SCMs should undergo screening of the whole neural axis. All possible causes of tethering should be addressed at the time of the surgery. The new clinically relevant classification is proposed with impetus on subclassifying type I SCM. Classification will aid in surgical planning and complication avoidance. Type Ia SCM carries the possibility of good surgical outcomes, and type Id carries higher risk of postoperative neurological deterioration.

References

1. Dias MS, Walker ML. The embryogenesis of complex dysraphic malformations: a disorder of gastrulation? Pediatr Neurosurg 1992;18(5–6):229–253
2. Sinha S, Agarwal D, Mahapatra AK. Split cord malformations: an experience of 203 cases. Childs Nerv Syst 2006;22(1):3–7
3. Guthkelch AN. Diastematomyelia with median septum. Brain 1974;97(4):729–742
4. Pang D, Dias MS, Ahab-Barmada M. Split cord malformation: part I—a unified theory of embryogenesis for double spinal cord malformations. Neurosurgery 1992;31(3):451–480
5. Pang D. Split cord malformation: part II—clinical syndrome. Neurosurgery 1992;31(3):481–500
6. Ailawadhi P, Mahapatra AK. An unusual case of spinal dysraphism with four splits including three posterior spurs. Pediatr Neurosurg 2011;47(5):372–375
7. Singh PK, Khandelwal A, Singh A, Ailawadhi P, Gupta D, Mahapatra AK. Long-segment type 1 split cord malformation with two-level split cord malformation and a single dural sac at the lower split. Pediatr Neurosurg 2011;47(3):227–229
8. Harwood-Nash DC, McHugh K. Diastematomyelia in 172 children: the impact of modern neuroradiology. Pediatr Neurosurg 1990–1991–1991;16(4-5):247–251
9. Chandra PS, Kamal R, Mahapatra AK. An unusual case of dorsally situated bony spur in a lumbar split cord malformation. Pediatr Neurosurg 1999;31(1):49–52
10. Alzhrani GA, Al-Jehani HM, Melançon D. Multi-level split cord malformation: do we need a new classification? J Clin Imaging Sci 2014;4:32
11. Kumar R, Singh SN, Bansal KK, Singh V. Comparative study of complex spina bifida and split cord malformation. Indian J Pediatr 2005;72(2):109–115
12. Ozturk E, Sonmez G, Mutlu H, et al. Split-cord malformation and accompanying anomalies. J Neuroradiol 2008;35(3):150–156
13. Higashida T, Sasano M, Sato H, Sekido K, Ito S. Myelomeningocele associated with split cord malformation type I: three case reports. Neurol Med Chir (Tokyo) 2010;50(5):426–430

14. Kumar R, Singh SN. Spinal dysraphism: trends in northern India. Pediatr Neurosurg 2003;38(3): 133–145

15. Kumar R, Bansal KK, Chhabra DK. Occurrence of split cord malformation in meningomyelocele: complex spina bifida. Pediatr Neurosurg 2002;36(3):119–127

16. Akiyama K, Nishiyama K, Yoshimura J, Mori H, Fujii Y. A case of split cord malformation associated with myeloschisis. Childs Nerv Syst 2007;23(5):577–580

17. Yamanaka T, Hashimoto N, Sasajima H, Mineura K. A case of diastematomyelia associated with myeloschisis in a hemicord. Pediatr Neurosurg 2001;35(5):253–256

18. Rowley VB, Johnson AJ. Lumbar split cord malformation with lateral hemimyelomeningocele and associated Chiari II malformation and other visceral and osseous anomalies: a case report. J Comput Assist Tomogr 2009;33(6):923–926

19. Parmar H, Patkar D, Shah J, Maheshwari M. Diastematomyelia with terminal lipomyelocystocele arising from one hemicord: case report. Clin Imaging 2003;27(1):41–43

20. Khandelwal A, Tandon V, Mahapatra AK. An unusual case of 4 level spinal dysraphism: Multiple composite type 1 and type 2 split cord malformation, dorsal myelocystocele and hydrocephalous. J Pediatr Neurosci 2011;6(1):58–61

21. Gupta DK, Mahapatra AK. Terminal myelocystoceles: a series of 17 cases. J Neurosurg 2005; 103(4, Suppl):344–352

22. Jaiswal AK, Mahapatra AK. Terminal myelocystocele. J Clin Neurosci 2005;12(3):249–252

23. Morioka T, Hashiguchi K, Yoshida F, et al. Neurosurgical management of occult spinal dysraphism associated with OEIS complex. Childs Nerv Syst 2008;24(6):723–729

24. Emmez H, Tokgöz N, Dogulu F, Yilmaz MB, Kale A, Baykaner MK. Seven distinct coexistent cranial and spinal anomalies. Pediatr Neurosurg 2006;42(5):316–319

25. Avcu S, Köseoğlu MN, Bulut MD, Ozen O, Unal O. The association of tethered cord, syringomyelia, diastometamyelia, spinal epidermoid, spinal lipoma and dermal sinus tract in a child. JBR-BTR 2010;93(6):305–307

26. Solanki GA, Evans J, Copp A, Thompson DN. Multiple coexistent dysraphic pathologies. Childs Nerv Syst 2003;19(5–6):376–379

27. Maiti TK, Bhat DI, Devi BI, Sampath S, Mahadevan A, Shankar SK. Teratoma in split cord malformation: an unusual association: a report of two cases with a review of the literature. Pediatr Neurosurg 2010;46(3):238–241

28. Dwarakanath S, Suri A, Garg A, Mahapatra AK, Mehta VS. Adult complex spinal dysraphism with situs inversus totalis: a rare association and review. Spine 2005;30(8):E225–E228

29. Tubbs RS, Oakes WJ. Adult complex spinal dysraphism with situs inversus totalis: a rare association and review. Spine 2005;30(20):2356

30. Naik V, Mahapatra AK, Gupta C, Suri V. Complex split cord malformation with mediastinal extension of a teratoma and simultaneous ventral and dorsal bony spur splitting the cord. Pediatr Neurosurg 2010;46(5):368–372

31. Shieh C, Lam CH. A lateral cervical lipomyelomeningocele associated with diplomyelia. Pediatr Neurosurg 2006;42(6):399–403

32. Mahapatra AK, Gupta DK. Split cord malformations: a clinical study of 254 patients and a proposal for a new clinical-imaging classification. J Neurosurg 2005; 103(6, Suppl):531–536

33. Gupta DK, Mahapatra AK. Proposal for a new clinicoradiological classification of type I split-cord malformations: a prospective study of 25 cases. Pediatr Neurosurg 2006;42(6):341–346

34. Borkar SA, Mahapatra AK. Split cord malformations: a two years experience at AIIMS. Asian J Neurosurg 2012;7(2):56–60

35. Warder DE. Tethered cord syndrome and occult spinal dysraphism. Neurosurg Focus 2001;10(1):e1

36. Gower DJ, Del Curling O, Kelly DL Jr, Alexander E Jr. Diastematomyelia—a 40-year experience. Pediatr Neurosci 1988;14(2):90–96

CHAPTER 4

Split Cord Malformations Type I

Shweta Kedia, Rajesh Meena, and Ashok K. Mahapatra

Table of Contents

- Introduction 31

- Anatomy and Classification 31

- Inheritance 32

- Clinical Presentation 32

- Imaging 34

- Management 35

- Complications 37

- Outcome 37

Split Cord Malformations Type I

Shweta Kedia, Rajesh Meena, and Ashok K. Mahapatra

Introduction

The first mention of split cord malformation (SCM) type I was made for a 1,800-year-old cadaver with a butterfly-shaped vertebra at the thoracolumbar junction, which had a bony spur that divided the spinal canal into two.[1–4] However, Ollivier[5] has been rightly credited to have described diastematomyelia in 1837. The origin of this term is Greek: diastema synonym of cleft, and myelos for cord. In 1892, almost 55 years later, Hertwig used the term "diastematomyelia" for split spinal cord, each having an individual dural sac divided by a bony spur in the midline with a single set of dorsal as well as ventral nerve roots.[5]

SCM is considered a presentation of occult spinal dysraphism. It is present mostly in the pediatric population, but there are few cases reported in adults as well.[6,7] The literature suggests the incidence rate of 2 to 4 per 1,000 live births, but it may be misleading,[8] as it has a complex presentation and may not always be diagnosed correctly.[9–12] The female to male ratio is 1.5–1.3:1 and is suggestive of female preponderance.[9–13] The classical description of SCM type I is when the spinal cord is divided by a bony spur into two hemicords in the sagittal plane, each having their own central canal with dorsal and anterior horns and usually associated with a low-lying conus with thick or fatty filum.[8] These patients have varied degree of urological, musculoskeletal, and sensory system involvement with subtle or obvious cutaneous markers.

In this chapter, we shall discuss the anatomy, imaging, clinical presentation, management, and outcome of SCM type I. Embryogenesis has been discussed in chapter 2 in the book.

Anatomy and Classification

SCM has been commonly classified into two types: type I with an intervening bony or fibrocartilaginous spur dividing the neural tube into two with separate dural sheath, and type II, where there is a fibrous septum between two hemicords and a single dural sheath which encloses the split cord.[14]

Not all SCMs fit these descriptions precisely, and there has been several attempts to reclassify the SCM for a better anatomic understanding.[9] In their paper, Mahapatra et al have attempted to classify the SCM I into four subtypes. They studied the location and extent of the bone spur bifurcating the spinal cord and based on that they explained each subtype in surgical context.[9]

The bony spur extends in the anteroposterior direction and usually divides the canal with the cord into two almost equal halves, or at times the spur runs oblique in the axial plane, and this divides the spinal cord into asymmetrical halves, one of which is normal and the other abnormal, hypoplastic. The embryogenesis also supports this new classification. Type Ia SCM in this classification can be because of the endomesenchymal tract disappearing variably at the upper and lower portions after splitting the notochord and the neural plate. Primitive meninx induces bone formation in the center of the split. Likewise, in Type Ib, the endomesenchymal tract disappears caudally, while in Type Ic the endomesenchymal tract remained persistent at the lower pole. Type Id has wide, tight split with the bone septum straddling the bifurcation, and here the endomesenchymal tract remains persistent throughout. The MRI and the axial CT scan findings often correlate with this classification and help surgeons anticipate the intraoperative findings.[15]

The spur is most commonly observed in the lumbar area, but also has been reportedly observed in the cervical, lower thoracic, upper thoracic, and sacrum in decreasing order of frequency.[12]

It is not also unusual to find that the two hemicords continue as two different fila, but normally at the end of the spur, they join together to continue as a single filum. In the presence of two separate fila, one should think of composite SCMs and go through the imaging carefully.[16–18]

Inheritance

Most of the times, SCMs appear in isolation and does not show a familial pattern. Only four cases mentioned in the literature showed a hereditary pattern and all of them were in females.[19] No reports mention an affected parent and a child. However, again, these numbers may be misleading because of the rarity of reporting. Some authors did suggest an X-linked inheritance in a dominant fashion.

Unlike, the often-quoted risk incidence of 4% of having an affected child for parents with spinal dysraphism, it cannot be said for a parent with SCM.[20]

Clinical Presentation

The usual presentation is at the age of 2 to 4 years, with a second peak at adolescence at the time of rapid growth. With the advancement in the imaging, the age at diagnosis can range from the prenatal period to adulthood.[12,21–24]

The presenting symptoms can be divided into cutaneous stigmata, deformities in the lower limb/musculoskeletal system, and neurological deficits (**Box 4.1**).

Hypertrichosis is the most common skin manifestation.[25–31] Pang[25] in his paper on clinical presentation of split cord suggested that these cutaneous manifestations may result from minor aberrations occurring during the surface ectoderm development. It is not so commonly present in patients with myelomeningocele (MMC), as these aberrations are overshadowed by chaotic changes occurring in the surface ectoderm, which are also occasioned by the unneurulated neural plate. This theory has been supported by other authors as well.[31,32]

All the structural deformities that occur in patients with SCM type I makes it surgically challenging. Literature states that scoliosis may be seen in almost 30 to 60% of patients with SCM.[29,30] Also, conversely, 5% of patients with congenital scoliosis may have underlying SCM.[30,33–36] Higher the age of the child, more are the chances of scoliotic deformity (**Fig. 4.1**).

It has been observed that the presenting complaint of adults with SCM is usually back pain and sciatica, as a part of manifestation of tethered cord.[6,37] Occasionally, skin, musculoskeletal, or neurological

---

Box 4.1 List of clinical signs and symptomatology

Cutaneous findings
- Hypertrichosis.
- Capillary hemangioma.
- Hyperpigmentation.
- Dimple.
- Subcutaneous lipoma.

Orthopedic deformities
- Kyphoscoliosis.
- Unilateral lower limb atrophy.
- Pes echinovarus/cavus/valgus/calcaneovarus.
- Neurotrophic ulcers in foot.
- Spontaneous amputation of toes.

Neurological findings
- Low back pain.
- Paraparesis/paraplegia, monoparesis with or without bladder and bowel involvement.

Box 4.2 List of associations with SCM type I

Concurrent congenital associations
- Thick filum terminale.
- MMC.
- Hemimyelomeningocele/meningocele.
- MMC manqué.
- Dermal sinus tract.
- Teratoma.
- Dermoid cyst.
- Intradural arachnoid cyst.
- Occipital encephalocele.
- Craniosynostosis, and dural arteriovenous malformation of the posterior fossa.

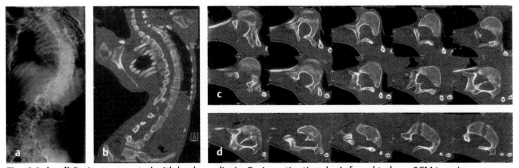

Fig. 4.1 (a–d) Patient presented with kyphoscoliosis. On investigation, he is found to have SCM type I.

abnormalities may also be present since childhood but were ignored.[33,38–41] Usually, trauma or strenuous exercise may lead to the precipitation of symptoms.[6] SCMs have been shown to be associated with the anomalies listed in **Box 4.2**.

The most common association is that of a thick filum terminale, which is responsible for tethered cord syndrome and should be specifically looked for preoperatively. The failure to notice and divide this leads to recurrence of symptoms because of tethering.[42,43] The bony split is 3 to 4 times more commonly seen with MMC and is present at or just cranial to the level of the defect. Emery and Lendon, in their paper, state that the incidence of SCM in MMC patients is around 78%.[44] Neurenteric cysts may also be found in conjunction with SCMs.[45–47]

Imaging

The available imaging modalities which help in diagnosing and planning surgery include X-ray, USG, CT, and MRI. Each has its own advantages and disadvantages.

The better prognosis of SCM makes it very important to diagnose it in utero and distinguish it from other kinds of spinal dysraphism. The first ever prenatal diagnosis of SCM was made by Williams, and now it has become quite common.[48] Literature now states in abundance the characteristic features of SCM (**Box 4.3**).

These criteria help diagnose SCM with a high specificity. The mean gestational age around which the diagnosis can be comfortably made is around 21.5 weeks (13–33 weeks).[49,50] Fetal MRI, although not commonly done, is another diagnostic tool. It is found to be more useful at a later gestational stage.[51] Along with imaging, amniotic fluid is assessed for acetyl-cholinesterase, and karyotyping may be done at the same time.[52]

In the postnatal period, MRI is the imaging of choice. The purpose of MRI is twofold in cases of SCM type I. First, it helps characterize the bony spur, its obliquity, and levels (**Fig. 4.2**). Second, it helps define the associated anomalies which may be otherwise missed.[53] Hence, the need to do a screening MRI. It is a noninvasive way of diagnosing hydromyelia and defining associated lesions. It is superior in determining tethered cord than CT and should always be looked for.

CT scan is superior to MRI in identifying the spur and its extent.[54,55] It also helps in visualizing the shape and direction. Reconstructed 3D CT scans with thin-slice has a positive detection rate close to 100%.

Based on the CT scan, it has been observed that these spurs are in the lumbar area in almost 50% of the patients, 27% in thoracolumbar and 23% in thoracic, and 1.5% in sacral or cervical.[45]

Plain X-ray films are extremely useful in picking up the bone deformities like kyphoscoliosis, bifid lamina, vertebral anomalies, and narrowing of the intervertebral disc space.[12,28,30] The prominent spinous process in the area of the bone spur is also a marker of SCM type I. The full sagittal profile is a must in patients with associated kyphoscoliosis.

Box 4.3 USG characteristics of SCM

- Wide spinal canal in the coronal plane.
- New echogenic focus traversing anteroposterior walls of the spinal canal in the axial plane.
- Skin and soft tissue abnormalities overlying the affected segment.
- Presence of echogenic foci in the posterior aspect of vertebral column.

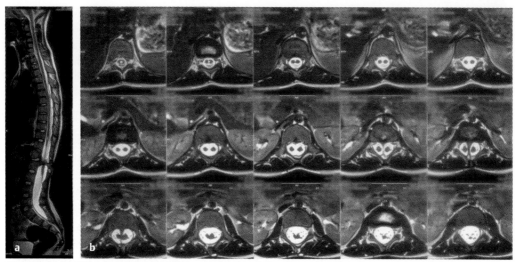

Fig. 4.2 (a, b) MRI is helpful in identifying the level and classifying the split. The angulation of the spur is nearly horizontal in this case. Also, note the level of conus ending at upper border of L3. Hydromyelia at D11 is also present. The axial scan shows Type Ia split as per Mahapatra's classification.

Management

The management of SCM involves surgical removal in a symptomatic patient. Even in asymptomatic patients, especially children, it should be surgically removed for the fear of neurological deterioration during growth spurt.

■ Timing of Surgery

It is controversial. SCM is progressive in nature.[56] Few authors recommend early prophylactic surgery in asymptomatic patients.[54,57–59] While few others consider it as a high-surgical risk and prefer to wait.[60] In the current era, authors have shifted into a more proactive approach and prefer to provide an early surgical removal in all the patients.[61,62]

■ Surgical Technique

Matson in 1950 described for the first time the surgical technique of the midline bone septum resection.[63] Moes in 1963 and Hendrick & Meacham in 1967 described the surgical steps and technical intricacies to achieve a good result.[64,65]

This surgery is technically demanding, and great care needs to be taken to avoid new deficits. A brief outline of the surgical technique followed by the authors in their institute is provided.

All patients receive general anesthesia (GA) in prone position. Motor evoked potential (MEP)/ somatosensory evoked potential (SSEP) monitoring is used intraoperatively. Although the associated cutaneous anomaly gives a good clue about the likely location of the spur is, it is a good practice to take the fluoroscopic guidance in cases of multilevel involvement.

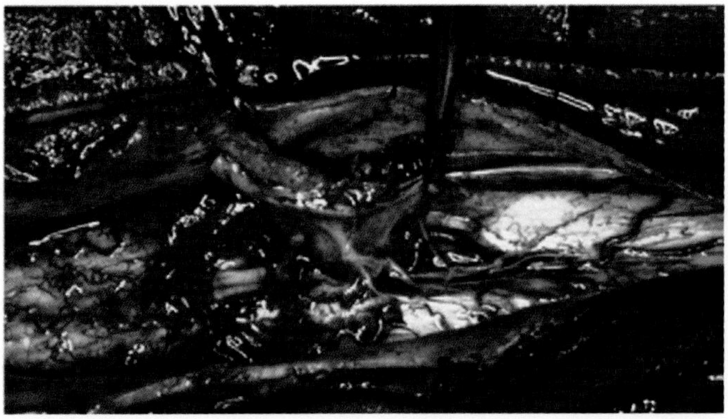

Fig. 4.3 Intraoperative imaging of SCM type I after opening the dural sac. The two separate dural sacs with the interdural portion of the bony spur are identifiable. The median nerve roots can be sacrificed.

The incision is placed in the midline centered over the prominent spinous process. Dissection is carried out to do a subperiosteal exposure of the spinous process and lamina. Laminotomy is preferred in children whereas laminectomy can be performed in adults. Care should be taken not to do en-bloc laminotomy, especially in dorsoventral spurs. The cutting drill is quite useful at this point but should be used cautiously. There is a high likelihood of injuring the cord at the level of the split, and therefore one should tread carefully. Diamond drill can be used in the last portion of the residual bony spur, under copious irrigation to prevent thermal damage to the cord.

The bony spur is identified and dissected meticulously subperiosteally and separated from the dura matter under microscope. It is removed extra durally as much as possible. Small arteries and veins may be present at the point of insertion of the spur on the vertebral body, which are coagulated using the bipolar forceps. It is important to ensure hemostasis at this level. The dural sac is now opened in an elliptical shape and joined to each other at either ends to obtain a single dural sac. The interdural portion of the spur can now be removed to obtain a flat posterior vertebral body (**Fig. 4.3**). Authors do not reconstruct the anterior dura usually, but some surgeons may prefer to do so. The lateral edges of the two dural sacs are sutured together using a nonresorbable suture in a continuous manner, preferably 5–0 Prolene, to make a single dural sac.

The last and the most important step is to identify the filum and detether it. Dura is then sutured to obtain a watertight closure, and the laminotomy is reconstructed. The muscle, fascia, and skin are closed in layers. Authors do not prefer to leave a subfascial drain, however, it may be kept when deemed necessary.

■ Postoperative Care

The patient is nursed in prone position for 48 hours and a close watch is kept on the wound. There are few patients who may show transient weakness and urinary retention because of intraoperative handling. Many of them recover in the follow-up period.

Authors generally do a follow-up MRI at 6 months interval. It is not uncommon to see the conus lying at the same level but is very rarely a cause of worry. Associated syrinx may also resolve.

Complications

Immediate complications include wound leak, neurological deficits, and blood loss. Early complications include pseudomeningocele, transient weakness, and wound infections. Late complications include bony regrowth. There are few cases of bony regrowth reported in literature. These patients present with delayed onset new deficits. It is recommended to repeat the CT as well as MRI of the suspected level. The hypothesis is that there are cell rests of meningeal residual polyvalent mesenchyma on the dura. The portion left behind in contact with the residual spur stimulates bone growth. Such patients do well with the re-exploration and reported to have significant neurological recovery after re-resection.[63,66,67]

Outcome

Often, patients who are neurologically intact preoperatively remain intact after surgery. As mentioned above, few of them may show a transient weakness, but show improvement to reach the baseline within 6 weeks. In his series of SCM I, Schijman actually divided his patients into three groups: (1) with neuro-orthopedic issues, (2) with only cutaneous manifestations, and (3) with associated other spinal dysraphism.[68] He observed that even those with prior deficits remained at their neurological baseline. Mahapatra et al, in their series, showed 50% of the patients did have neurological improvement postsurgery.[62] The ones with existing neurological deficits and scoliosis had the highest risk of deterioration.[61]

Pierre-Aurelien, in his study, reported neurological worsening in 5% of cases with almost 72% of the patients improved.[69] It is quite usual to see the motor deficits fare well almost after 6 months of surgery and may be expected to do so for almost 2 years. The authors did not observe any new onset urological complaints in their patients and almost 50% showed bladder recovery. However, the ones with associated meningomyelocele (MMC) had poor outcome. In authors' experience, the bladder recovery is quite unusual.

Based on his new proposed classification of SCM type I, Borkar et al suggest the ones with Type Id are most prone to persistent neurological worsening in the postoperative period.[62,70]

■ Scoliosis Management

The biggest concern in patients with SCM I is associated scoliosis. The scoliosis is associated with progression, especially when present with vertebral anomalies. It is a good practice to address the split first before going for scoliosis correction. This is a compromised cord. At the same time, Chiari malformation should be ruled out in these cases.[71,72]

Now, if the decision to correct the scoliosis has also been made, it is advisable to stage it to minimize the complication rates. This was in fact first recommended by Winter in 1974.[28] This way authors reduce the intraoperative time and the risk of infections. Considering these patients are going to need instrumentation for deformity correction, risk of infection is already high.[71,72]

References

1. Edelson JG, Nathan H, Arensburg B. Diastematomyelia: the "double-barrelled" spine. J Bone Joint Surg Br 1987;69(2):188–189
2. Lazareff JA. Neural Tube Defects. Singapore: World Scientific; 2011
3. Mathern GW, Peacock WJ. Diastematomyelia. In: Park TS, ed. Spinal Dysraphism. Contemporary Issues in Neurological Surgery. Boston: Blackwell Scientific; 1992:91–103
4. Saker E, Loukas M, Fisahn C, Oskouian RJ, Tubbs RS. Historical perspective of split cord malformations: a tale of two cords. Pediatr Neurosurg 2017;52(1):1–5
5. Hertwig O. Urmund und spina bifida. Arch Mikrosk Anat 1892;39:353–503
6. Russell NA, Benoit BG, Joaquin AJ. Diastematomyelia in adults. A review. Pediatr Neurosurg 1990–1991;16(4-5):252–257
7. Sheehan JP, Sheehan JM, Lopes MB, Jane JA Sr. Thoracic diastematomyelia with concurrent intradural epidermoid spinal cord tumor and cervical syrinx in an adult. Case report. J Neurosurg 2002; 97(2, Suppl):231–234
8. Jindal A, Mahapatra AK, Kamal R. Spinal dysraphism. Indian J Pediatr 1999;66(5):697–705
9. Gupta DK, Mahapatra AK. Proposal for a new clinicoradiological classification of type I split-cord malformations: a prospective study of 25 cases. Pediatr Neurosurg 2006;42(6):341–346
10. Gan YC, Sgouros S, Walsh AR, Hockley AD. Diastematomyelia in children: treatment outcome and natural history of associated syringomyelia. Childs Nerv Syst 2007;23(5):515–519
11. Börcek AÖ, Ocal O, Emmez H, Zinnuroğlu M, Baykaner MK. Split cord malformation: experience from a tertiary referral center. Pediatr Neurosurg 2012;48(5):291–298
12. Mahapatra AK. Split cord malformation: a study of 300 cases at AIIMS 1990–2006. J Pediatr Neurosci 2011;6(Suppl 1):S41–S45
13. Pang D, Dias MS, Ahab-Barmada M. Split cord malformation: Part I: A unified theory of embryogenesis for double spinal cord malformations. Neurosurgery 1992;31(3):451–480
14. Reigel DH, McLone DG. Tethered spinal cord. In: Cheek WR, Marlin AE, McLone DG, Reigel DH, Walker ML, eds. Pediatric Neurosurgery: Surgery of the Developing Nervous System. 3rd ed. Chapter 4. Philadelphia: Saunders; 1994:77–95
15. Prasad GL, Borkar SA, Satyarthee GD, Mahapatra AK. Split cord malformation with dorsally located bony spur: Report of four cases and review of literature. J Pediatr Neurosci 2012;7(3):167–170
16. Erşahin Y. Composite type of split cord malformations. Childs Nerv Syst 2002;18(3-4):111
17. Vaishya S, Kumarjain P. Split cord malformation: three unusual cases of composite split cord malformation. Childs Nerv Syst 2001;17(9):528–530
18. James CC, Lassman LP. Diastematomyelia and the tight filum terminale. J Neurol Sci 1970;10(2):193–196
19. Erşahin Y, Kitiş O, Oner K. Split cord malformation in two sisters. Pediatr Neurosurg 2002;37(5):240–244
20. Harper Peter S. Central Nervous System Disorders. Practical Genetic Counselling. London: Arnold; 2003:176
21. Anderson NG, Jordan S, MacFarlane MR, Lovell-Smith M. Diastematomyelia: diagnosis by prenatal sonography. AJR Am J Roentgenol 1994;163(4):911–914
22. Boulot P, Ferran JL, Charlier C, et al. Prenatal diagnosis of diastematomyelia. Pediatr Radiol 1993;23(1):67–68
23. Glasier CM, Chadduck WM, Leithiser RE Jr, Williamson SL, Seibert JJ. Screening spinal ultrasound in newborns with neural tube defects. J Ultrasound Med 1990;9(6):339–343
24. Sinha S, Agarwal D, Mahapatra AK. Split cord malformations: an experience of 203 cases. Childs Nerv Syst 2006;22(1):3–7

25. Pang D. Split cord malformation: Part II: Clinical syndrome. Neurosurgery 1992;31(3):481–500

26. Pang D. Split cord malformations. In: Pang D, ed. Disorders of the Pediatric Spine. New York: Raven Press; 1995:203–252

27. Miller A, Guille JT, Bowen JR. Evaluation and treatment of diastematomyelia. J Bone Joint Surg Am 1993;75(9):1308–1317

28. Winter RB, Haven JJ, Moe JH, Lagaard SM. Diastematomyelia and congenital spine deformities. J Bone Joint Surg Am 1974;56(1):27–39

29. Hilal SK, Marton D, Pollack E. Diastematomyelia in children. Radiographic study of 34 cases. Radiology 1974;112(3):609–621

30. Hood RW, Riseborough EJ, Nehme AM, Micheli LJ, Strand RD, Neuhauser EB. Diastematomyelia and structural spinal deformities. J Bone Joint Surg Am 1980;62(4):520–528

31. Humphreys RP, Hendrick EB, Hoffman HJ. Diastematomyelia. Clin Neurosurg 1983;30:436–456

32. Erşahin Y, Mutluer S, Kocaman S, Demirtaş E. Split spinal cord malformations in children. J Neurosurg 1998;88(1):57–65

33. Wolf AL, Tubman DE, Seljeskog EL. Diastematomyelia of the cervical spinal cord with tethering in an adult. Neurosurgery 1987;21(1):94–98

34. Keim HA, Greene AF. Diastematomyelia and scoliosis. J Bone Joint Surg Am 1973;55(7):1425–1435

35. Louw JA, Roos MF. Diastematomyelia without a median septum in congenital scoliosis. A report of 2 cases. S Afr Med J 1987;72(6):433–434

36. McMaster MJ. Occult intraspinal anomalies and congenital scoliosis. J Bone Joint Surg Am 1984;66(4):588–601

37. Pang D, Wilberger JE Jr. Tethered cord syndrome in adults. J Neurosurg 1982;57(1):32–47

38. Dias MS, Walker ML. The embryogenesis of complex dysraphic malformations: a disorder of gastrulation? Pediatr Neurosurg 1992;18(5-6):229–253

39. English WJ, Maltby GL. Diastematomyelia in adults. J Neurosurg 1967;27(3):260–264

40. Freeman LW. Late symptoms from diastematomyelis. J Neurosurg 1961;18:538–541

41. List J, Stendel R, Rudolph KH, Brock M. [A case of diastematomyelia (split cord malformation type I) with clinical manifestation in adulthood]. Zentralbl Neurochir 1994;55(4):212–217

42. Guthkelch AN, Hoffmann GT. Tethered spinal cord in association with diastematomyelia. Surg Neurol 1981;15(5):352–354

43. Barutcuoglu M, Selcuki M, Selcuki D, et al. Cutting filum terminale is very important in split cord malformation cases to achieve total release. Childs Nerv Syst 2015;31(3):425–432

44. Emery JL, Lendon RG. The local cord lesion in neurospinal dysraphism (meningomyelocele). J Pathol 1973;110(1):83–96

45. Birch BD, McCormick PC. High cervical split cord malformation and neurenteric cyst associated with congenital mirror movements: case report. Neurosurgery 1996;38(4):813–815, discussion 815–816

46. Muthukumar N, Arunthathi J, Sundar V. Split cord malformation and neurenteric cyst—case report and a theory of embryogenesis. Br J Neurosurg 2000;14(5):488–492

47. Habibi Z, Hanaei S, Nejat F. Sacral extradural arachnoid cyst in association with split cord malformation. Spine J 2016;16(9):1109–1115

48. Williams RA, Barth RA. In utero sonographic recognition of diastematomyelia. AJR Am J Roentgenol 1985;144(1):87–88

49. Li SL, Luo G, Norwitz ER, et al. Prenatal diagnosis of diastematomyelia: a case report and review of the literature. J Clin Ultrasound 2012;40(5):301–305

50. Has R, Yuksel A, Buyukkurt S, Kalelioglu I, Tatli B. Prenatal diagnosis of diastematomyelia: presentation of eight cases and review of the literature. Ultrasound Obstet Gynecol 2007;30(6):845–849

51. Struben H, Visca E, Holzgreve W, et al. Prenatal diagnosis of diastematomyelia and tethered cord – a case report and review of the literature. Ultraschall Med 2008;29(1):72–76

52. Kutuk MS, Ozgun MT, Tas M, Poyrazoglu HG, Yikilmaz A. Prenatal diagnosis of split cord malformation by ultrasound and fetal magnetic resonance imaging: case report and review of the literature. Childs Nerv Syst 2012;28(12):2169–2172

53. Khandelwal A, Tandon V, Mahapatra AK. An unusual case of 4 level spinal dysraphism: Multiple composite type 1 and type 2 split cord malformation, dorsal myelocystocele and hydrocephalous. J Pediatr Neurosci 2011;6(1):58–61

54. Cardoso M, Keating RF. Neurosurgical management of spinal dysraphism and neurogenic scoliosis. Spine 2009;34(17):1775–1782

55. Cheng B, Li FT, Lin L. Diastematomyelia: a retrospective review of 138 patients. J Bone Joint Surg Br 2012;94(3):365–372

56. Goldberg C, Fenelon G, Blake NS, Dowling F, Regan BF. Diastematomyelia: a critical review of the natural history and treatment. Spine 1984;9(4):367–372

57. Jindal A, Mahapatra AK. Split cord malformations—a clinical study of 48 cases. Indian Pediatr 2000;37(6):603–607

58. Akay KM, Izci Y, Baysefer A, Timurkaynak E. Split cord malformation in adults. Neurosurg Rev 2004;27(2):99–105

59. Proctor MR, Scott RM. Long-term outcome for patients with split cord malformation. Neurosurg Focus 2001;10(1):e5

60. Jamil M, Bannister CM. A report of children with spinal dysraphism managed conservatively. Eur J Pediatr Surg 1992;2(Suppl 1):26–28

61. Lewandrowski KU, Rachlin JR, Glazer PA. Diastematomyelia presenting as progressive weakness in an adult after spinal fusion for adolescent idiopathic scoliosis. Spine J 2004;4(1):116–119

62. Mahapatra AK, Gupta DK. Split cord malformations: a clinical study of 254 patients and a proposal for a new clinical-imaging classification. J Neurosurg 2005; 103(6, Suppl):531–536

63. Matson DD, Woods RP, Campbell JB, Ingraham FD. Diastematomyelia (congenital clefts of the spinal cord); diagnosis and surgical treatment. Pediatrics 1950;6(1):98–112

64. Moes CAF, Hendrick EB. Diastematomyelia. J Pediatr 1963;63(2):238–248

65. Meacham WF. Surgical treatment of diastematomyelia. J Neurosurg 1967;27(1):78–85

66. Pang D, Parrish RG. Regrowth of diastematomyelic bone spur after extradural resection. Case report. J Neurosurg 1983;59(5):887–890

67. Gupta DK, Ahmed S, Garg K, Mahapatra AK. Regrowth of septal spur in split cord malformation. Pediatr Neurosurg 2010;46(3):242–244

68. Schijman E. Split spinal cord malformations: report of 22 cases and review of the literature. Childs Nerv Syst 2003;19(2):96–103

69. Beuriat PA, Di Rocco F, Szathmari A, Mottolese C. Management of split cord malformation in children: the Lyon experience. Childs Nerv Syst 2018;34(5):883–891

70. Borkar SA, Mahapatra AK. Split cord malformations: a two years experience at AIIMS. Asian J Neurosurg 2012;7(2):56–60

71. Feng F, Shen J, Zhang J, et al. Clinical outcomes of different surgical strategy for patients with congenital scoliosis and type I split cord malformation. Spine 2016;41(16):1310–1316

72. Hui H, Tao H-R, Jiang X-F, Fan HB, Yan M, Luo ZJ. Safety and efficacy of 1-stage surgical treatment of congenital spinal deformity associated with split spinal cord malformation. Spine 2012;37(25):2104–2113

CHAPTER 5

Split Cord Malformations Type II

Amol Raheja, Tarang K. Vora, and Ashok K. Mahapatra

Table of Contents

- Introduction 43

- Embryogenesis and Histopathology 43

- Clinical Presentation 45

- Diagnostic Imaging and Radiological Workup 46

- Principles of Management 47

- Conclusions 48

Split Cord Malformations Type II

Amol Raheja, Tarang K. Vora, and Ashok K. Mahapatra

Introduction

Split cord malformation (SCM) is the currently acceptable nomenclature for any patient with double spinal cords. The unique morphology of SCM acquired by each patient depends on three embryogenetic fates of the endomesenchymal tract: (1) variable extent to which endomesenchymal tract persists; (2) the embryo's ability to heal around endomesenchymal tract; and (3) the cumulative destiny of dislocated midline mesoderm and endoderm.[1,2]

As per Pang's classification, SCM is further subclassified into type I/II, based on median septum characteristics and dural tube status surrounding the two hemicords.[1,2] SCM type I houses each hemicord in its own dural tube, which are separated by a rigid osseocartilaginous midline septum. On the contrary, SCM type II consists of a single dural tube housing two hemicords separated by a fibrous median septum, which is nonrigid[1,2] (**Fig. 5.1**). This currently acceptable classification helps subdivide SCM cases preoperatively, based on the radiological imaging, and further plan their surgical management and risk assessment accordingly.[1,3,4] This chapter has been conceptualized to understand the embryogenesis, clinical presentation, diagnostic imaging, radiological workup, decision-making process, and surgical strategy in management of individuals with SCM type II.

Embryogenesis and Histopathology

In contrast to SCM type I, pathogenesis of type II malformation involves lack of precursor cells' recruitment from meninx primitiva during the mesenchymal investment period over the abnormal fistula (accessory neurenteric canal), it is possibly attributable to the completion of endomesenchymal tract prior to the appearance of definite meninx primitiva (day 30).[2] Hence, the development of midline mesenchymal components will be much less complex in type II malformation, where only a thin fibrous septum is formed between the two hemicords. Moreover, the fibrous septum of type II SCM is anatomically located at the caudal extent of the split, and is usually oriented obliquely in such a fashion that its dural attachment is almost always caudal to its hemicords attachment.[2,3,5,6] The explanation for this observation is that relatively more compliant endomesenchymal tract in SCM type II presumably renders the hemicords with slightly higher degree of freedom for vertical movement as compared to SCM type I. More permissive and pliable transfixation of the neural tube by the endomesenchymal tract in SCM type II probably also accounts for lower extent of "splitting" of the cord seen in SCM type II when compared to SCM type I.[2,3,5,6] The fact that majority of type II SCM cases have intact overlying skin over the split cords implies that the cutaneous ectoderm closed the dorsal opening of fistulous neurenteric canal and formed intact skin in the early stage of its embryogenesis. However, the involvement of surface ectoderm by dorsal endomesenchymal tract can get manifested in the form of hypertrichosis,

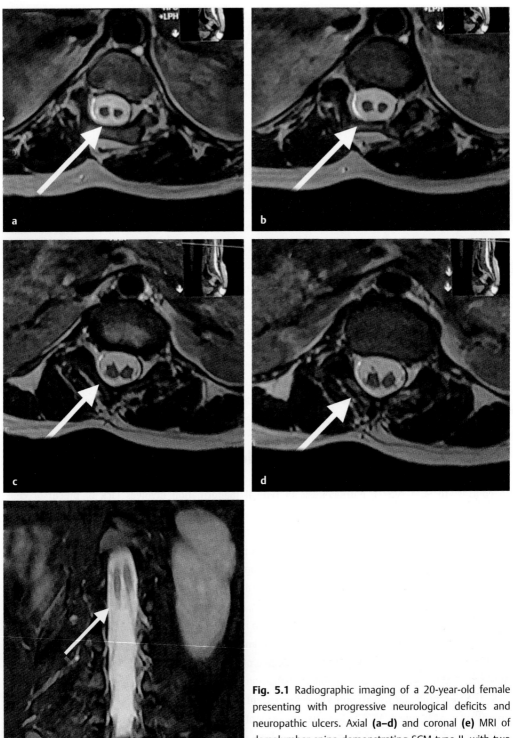

Fig. 5.1 Radiographic imaging of a 20-year-old female presenting with progressive neurological deficits and neuropathic ulcers. Axial **(a–d)** and coronal **(e)** MRI of dorsolumbar spine demonstrating SCM type II, with two hemicords lying within the single dural tube (marked by arrow). There is no bony spur seen in the median septum separating and tethering the two hemicords.

capillary hemangioma, etc.[2,3,5,6] A more infrequent association of open myelomeningocele and SCM can be occasionally seen, although the exact embryogenetic mechanism accounting for such an association is not known.[2,3,5,6]

Pluripotent cells from endomesenchymal tract could develop into multiple discrete tissues. Ersahin[3] demonstrated that pathological specimens from median septa of SCM patients reveal lymphoid tissue, blood vessels, dermoid cysts, tubular epithelia, muscle tissue, ganglion cells, fetal renal tissue and, rarely, teratomas in addition to osseocartilaginous tissue seen in SCM. The hypothesis for the presence of displaced neural crest cells in the median fibrous septum of SCM type II stems from the histological evidence of presence of ganglion cells, suggesting that the "extra" nerve roots in median septum are essentially the central processes of neural crest cells entrapped by the endomesenchymal tract.[2,3] Intestinal duplication or neurenteric cyst, endodermal remnants of endomesenchymal tract, may be rarely associated with SCM type II.[2,3] Persistence of ventral and dorsal endomesenchymal tract leads to differential association of dermoids, intestinal malrotation, and dermal sinus tract with SCM type II. The theory of ectoendodermal adhesion and endomesenchymal tract is further supported by the presence of variable degree of ectodermal, mesenchymal, and endodermal structures detected from the median septa.[2,3]

Clinical Presentation

SCM is noticed in approximately 20% of children with neural tube defects.[1,4,6] Neurological deficits are proportionately distributed across both SCM types I and II. In a large series of 300 SCM patients by Mahapatra,[4] it was demonstrated that 60% of patients had cutaneous marker and 80% had scoliosis or lower limb deformities, which act as surrogate markers for underlying SCM. The most frequently associated cutaneous marker with SCM type II is hypertrichosis, with an incidence varying from 20 to 55%.[1,3,4,6] Majority of SCMs are seen in lumbosacral region, followed by dorsal region, and only rare instances of cervical cord tethering by SCM type II has been reported in the literature. Therefore, a strong clinical suspicion is paramount in timely diagnosis of cervical SCMs, which if left untreated may lead to hand dysfunction apart from spastic legs.[1,3,4,6] Their frequent association with Klippel-Feil syndrome (KFS) and associated phenotypes in the neck justifies a screening MRI to rule out underlying occult SCM or other associated spinal dysraphic elements.[1,3,4,6] In a series of 131 SCM patients, Ersahin[3] noted that the patients with orthopedic deformities and neurological deficits were significantly older and were symptomatic for longer duration than those without deficits, probably owing to progressive tethering of the spinal cord. All such patients should be explored and intervened surgically once diagnosed, especially before the onset of permanent neurological and orthopedic sequelae.

Tethered cord syndrome symptomatology is also evident in SCM type II.[1,4–8] Gait disturbance is the most common presenting complaint in children, followed by pain and progressive foot and spinal deformities. On the contrary, adults often present with severe dysesthetic pain in the perineum and legs, followed by sensory and motor deficits.[1,4–8] Delayed bowel and bladder involvement is also a common part of clinical symptomatology. Asymmetric splitting of spinal cord by median septum oriented in an oblique fashion into a large "major" hemicord and a small "minor" hemicord may lead to bilateral functional discrepancy.[1,4–8] The proposed hypothesis behind such an observation is that the oblique course of the fistulous tract has not only divided the neural cell population of segmented neurons unevenly for the two halves of the body but also seems to have deprived the minor cord of adequate ascending and descending axons.[1,4-8] Pathological specimens have also corroborated this theory by demonstrating rudimentary anterior and posterior gray horns and thin disorganized white funiculi in the minor hemicords. On the contrary, major hemicords have been shown to acquire three gray columns of robust neurons. Besides, presence of syrinx can also be asymmetric, which may lead to worse neurological function on the affected side. A constellation of systemic anomalies is commonly associated with patients afflicted with SCM, which include urogenital anomalies, cardiovascular anomalies, and anorectal malformations.[9] Other reported associations include eventration of the diaphragm and situs invertus.[4,6,10]

Diagnostic Imaging and Radiological Workup

Given the fact that there is a high probability of irreversible and progressive neurological deterioration if a SCM is unrecognized, it is arguably justified to screen every child with surrogate markers of spinal dysraphism with an MRI.[1,3] If a SCM is identified, it should be treated and explored, because its deleterious effect on the spinal cord is independent of the state of treated neural placode under consideration.[1,3] MRI is the diagnostic imaging of choice for evaluation and planning management of SCM in the present era, although CT myelogram has also been invaluable in providing detailed topographic anatomy of the midline septum and its relationship with neural and vascular structures, especially few decades ago.[1,3,4,6] However, CT myelogram has the disadvantages of use of ionizing radiation, lumbar puncture and general anesthesia (GA) for young children. Routine workup of patients with suspected spinal dysraphism should include an MRI of the suspected site and screening MRI of the whole spine and brain to exclude any associated Chiari malformation, hydrocephalus or multisite spinal dysraphism.[1,3,4,6] Besides, any associated anomalies like lipoma, neurenteric cyst, dermoid/epidermoid tumor, thick/fatty filum, etc., can also be picked with these scans. Ultrasonography of abdomen is part of additional systemic workup for these patients, as it can find associated congenital anomalies. Urodynamic study on the other hand provides crucial clues toward early onset bladder involvement in patients with spinal dysraphism.[1,3,4,6] Renal scans may also be required in a certain subset of patients where glomerular filtration rate assessment is required to ascertain the degree of renal damage. Similarly, echocardiography is pivotal to rule out associated cardiac anomalies.

One of the constant features in type II SCM patients is that the fibrous septum is obliquely oriented with its neural attachment always rostral than its dural attachment, and a similar orientation of the associated myelomeningocele manqué.[1,3,4,6] These findings are attributed to the differential growth rates of developing vertebral column and neural tube after its preceding transfixation by the endomesenchymal tract. However, in many instances, fibrous septum can be radiologically inappreciable, although its presence can be confirmed intraoperatively in many of them. Barson[11] and others[12,13] have shown that the usual ascent of spinal cord continues postnatally till at least 1 year of age. Hence, as expected, children younger than 1 year of age tend to have significantly shorter split length as compared to those over 1 year of age at diagnosis. It has also been documented that cervical cord ascent relative to the adjacent vertebral column is less than that found in thoracolumbar segments which, in turn, corroborates with the shorter split length in cervical region as opposed to transfixation in lumbar region.[12,13] The incidence of SCM in open spinal dysraphism is higher than what was earlier expected, especially in the setting of right-left functional discrepancy of the lower limbs or if the spinal-neurological level does not correspond to the site of myelomeningocele sac.[1,4] These patients should also specifically undergo screening MRI of whole spine to rule out an associated SCM, as it may have significant bearing on surgical planning and patient outcome.

Principles of Management

Type II SCM, akin to type I SCM, is also considered to be a tethering lesion by virtue of tethering of hemicords via median fibrous septum which, in turn, is firmly inserted onto dural sac.[1,4] Tethering of median septum in SCM type II is released by simply excising the median fibrous septum after cauterizing the central vessels and dividing the nonfunctional paramedian roots. Early intervention to release tethering elements in SCM type II is the treatment of choice for symptomatic patients.[1,4] On the contrary, there is less convincing evidence in the literature for asymptomatic tethered cord patients with type II SCM, especially in adult patients.[1,7] In pediatric age group, many clinicians do tend to refer the children for prophylactic surgery; however, most adults are referred for treatment only after symptomatology ensues.[1,7] It is however advisable to operate on asymptomatic adult patients, especially who lead a physically active lifestyle, since trauma can precipitate acute neurological deterioration.[1,3,7] On the other hand, older asymptomatic adults living a sedentary lifestyle can possibly be offered conservative management. Surgical treatment offers best relief for pain, in general, and still remains the most common indication for surgery, especially among adult patients with SCM type II.[1,3,7] Sensorimotor deficits, on the other hand, are the next best responder; however, only recent onset deficits tend to improve. Finally, bowel bladder involvement is expected to improve in approximately 40% of patients, although another fraction of patients may experience stabilization of their previously progressive bladder/bowel symptoms.[1,3,7] On the contrary, progressive foot deformity may still ensue despite adequate detethering of the cord, which is attributed to irreversible osseoligamentous changes that are no longer affected by the existing neurological status. All the tethering lesions should be operated in same session, especially in a top-down approach, in order to prevent inadvertent and undue stretching of spinal cord after releasing lower tethering elements.[1,3,4,6,7] Laminotomy should be performed at the caudal end of split segment, as the base of fibrous spur is usually seen at the same anatomical location.[1,3,4,6,7]

In a series of 300 patients with SCM (55% were SCM type II) encountered over a period of 16 years, Mahapatra[4] demonstrated that overall improvement was noticed in 50% patients and stabilization in 44% cases, while 3% patients each had transient and permanent neurological deterioration. They recommended prophylactic surgery for even asymptomatic cases, as none of the patients developed postoperative neurological deficits and had an uneventful follow-up period.[4] In Pang's series of 18 SCM II patients, only five type II fibrous septae were demonstrated using radiological imaging preoperatively, although a fibrous septum was demonstrated to tether hemicords in each and every type II patient intraoperatively.[1,2] They argued quite ardently that all type II SCMs should be surgically explored, even if imaging studies does not reveal a definite median septum. Besides, they commented that the entire neuraxis should be evaluated to look for other accompanying tethering lesions, which may also require surgical exploration. Neurological status, generally, either improves or stabilizes after surgical exploration of type II SCM.[1] They observed three patterns of nonrigid septum based on its extent, anatomical relationship with the hemicords, and pattern of tethering.[1,2] Presence of central blood vessels in these fibrous septa is a constant feature either as parasagittal vessels or marginal artery.[1,2] They concluded that every SCM type II is a bonafide tethering lesion despite the fact that only nonrigid fibrous or fibrovascular septum is present between the two hemicords. In 2001, Pang et al[1] described ventral tethering in a series of 11 patients (21%) among 52 patients with type II SCM based upon their operative findings. They described four categories of ventral septa: (1) pure ventral intradural, (2) complete dorsoventral intradural septa, (3) dorsoventral septa continuous with an associated dermal sinus tract, and (4) ventral or complete septa continuous with the ventral intestinal bands causing intestinal malrotation or diverticulum. Based on these findings, they hypothesized that patients with dermal sinus tracts and intestinal malformations should be actively explored for ventral tethering elements in SCM type II patients.

Conclusions

SCM type II consists of a single dural tube housing two hemicords, separated by a fibrous median septum, which is nonrigid. Routine workup of patients with suspected spinal dysraphism should include an MRI of the suspected site and screening MRI of the whole spine and brain to exclude any associated Chiari malformation, hydrocephalus or multisite spinal dysraphism. Type II SCM, akin to type I SCM, is also considered to be a tethering lesion by virtue of tethering of hemicords via median fibrous septum which, in turn, is firmly inserted onto dural sac. Tethering of median septum in SCM type II is released by simply excising the median fibrous septum after cauterizing the central vessels and dividing the nonfunctional paramedian roots. Early intervention to release tethering elements in SCM type II is the treatment of choice for symptomatic patients. On the contrary, there is less convincing evidence in the literature for asymptomatic tethered cord patients with type II SCM, especially in adult patients.

References

1. Pang D. Split cord malformation: part II—clinical syndrome. Neurosurgery 1992;31(3):481–500
2. Pang D, Dias MS, Ahab-Barmada M. Split cord malformation: part I—a unified theory of embryogenesis for double spinal cord malformations. Neurosurgery 1992;31(3):451–480
3. Erşahin Y. Split cord malformation types I and II: a personal series of 131 patients. Childs Nerv Syst 2013;29(9):1515–1526
4. Mahapatra AK. Split cord malformation: a study of 300 cases at AIIMS 1990-2006. J Pediatr Neurosci 2011;6(Suppl 1):S41–S45
5. Jindal A, Mahapatra AK. Split cord malformations: a clinical study of 48 cases. Indian Pediatr 2000;37(6):603–607
6. Mahapatra AK, Gupta DK. Split cord malformations: a clinical study of 254 patients and a proposal for a new clinical-imaging classification. J Neurosurg 2005;103(6, Suppl):531–536
7. Pang D, Wilberger JE Jr. Tethered cord syndrome in adults. J Neurosurg 1982;57(1):32–47
8. Sinha S, Agarwal D, Mahapatra AK. Split cord malformations: an experience of 203 cases. Childs Nerv Syst 2006;22(1):3–7
9. Ozturk E, Sonmez G, Mutlu H, et al. Split-cord malformation and accompanying anomalies. J Neuroradiol 2008;35(3):150–156
10. Jindal A, Kansal S, Mahapatra AK. Split cord malformation with partial eventration of the diaphragm: case report. J Neurosurg 2000; 93(2, Suppl):309–311

11. Barson AJ. The vertebral level of termination of the spinal cord during normal and abnormal development. J Anat 1970;106(Pt 3):489–497

12. Barry A. A quantitative study of the prenatal changes in angulation of the spinal nerves. Anat Rec 1956;126(1):97–110

13. Barry JF, Harwood-Nash DC, Fitz CR, Byrd SE, Boldt DW. Metrizamide in pediatric myelography. Radiology 1977;124(2):409–418

Dorsal Spur

Sachin A. Borkar, Mohit Agrawal, and Ashok K. Mahapatra

Table of Contents

- Introduction 53
- Embryology 53
- Demography 54
- Clinical Features 54
- Imaging Studies 57
- Treatment 57
- Patient Outcome 58
- Conclusion 58

Dorsal Spur

Sachin A. Borkar, Mohit Agrawal, and Ashok K. Mahapatra

Introduction

Split cord malformation (SCM) is a congenital anomaly of the spinal cord, wherein there is splitting of the spinal cord over part of its length to form two neural tubes. The etiopathogenesis of this condition was unknown before Pang et al proposed their theory of "unified embryogenesis."[1-3] They described two varieties of SCM—type I which has a rigid bony septum between two hemicords, each within its own dural tube, and type II SCM comprising two hemicords in a single dural sac separated by a fibrous septum. This midline osseocartilaginous septum was described to always arise from the ventrally placed vertebral body. It was in 1999 when Chandra et al[4] described a new entity where the midline septum was seen to arise from the dorsal arch of the vertebrae. They named this as a dorsal spur.

Embryology

The earliest recognition of SCM as an abnormality was made by Ollivier in 1837 when he coined the term "diastematomyelia."[5] He described a spinal cord divided into two sleeves separated by a sagittal bony or fibrous spur. Bruce et al advised the use of the term diastematomyelia to only describe a spinal cord split by a midline bony spur. They proposed the term "diplomyelia" for true doubling of the cord without a spur.[6] These were just anatomical descriptions of the condition without elaborating on the etiopathogenesis of the condition. Feller and Stenberg were the first to indicate the embryological basis of this condition as a persistence of the midline cell rest and formation of a notochordal cleft.[7] Since then, several theories have been proposed in order to explain the genesis of SCM like the hydromyelic theory by Gardner in which he proposed that cerebrospinal fluid (CSF) causes the rupture of the neural tube, causing a split.[8] Primary mesodermal abnormality theory was advocated by Lichtenstein,[9] while Hendrick proposed the accessory neurenteric canal hypothesis.[10] Others proposed the mesodermal invasion of the neural tube.[11-13]

All these theories were laid to rest when Pang et al in 1992 proposed a unified theory of embryogenesis and recommended that the term "SCM" be used for all double spinal cords.[1-3] This theory essentially stated that a single error occurs at the time of closure of the primitive neurenteric canal, which leads to the persistent communication between the yolk sac and amnion through an "accessory neurenteric canal." This allows for a continued contact between the ectoderm and endoderm within the spinal canal. Subsequent mesenchymal infiltration and the timing of the formation of the endomesenchymal tract determines whether the neural tube splits into two separate hemicords each with their own dural sac with an intervening fibrocartilaginous or bony septum (diastematomyelia) or into two hemicords housed in a single dural sac with a fibrous septum dividing the two (diplomyelia). The important point to note here is that the development of the midline septum was described to always occur from a ventral direction, from the region of the vertebral body toward the posterior elements, splitting the canal in the middle. Chandra et al challenged this unified theory in 1999, when they described the entity known as dorsal spur.[4] They described a spur attached to a hypertrophied posterior arch (HPA), without any ventral attachment, thus contradicting the unified theory proposed by Pang et al. To explain this unusual finding, the authors proposed two possible hypotheses. The first was that during the process of abnormal migration of the meninx primitiva cells in between the split spinal cords, a sizable portion might get disconnected from the ventral tract and thus start accumulating dorsally. This abnormal mass would explain the formation of a dorsal spur with HPA. The second proposition was that the cells of meninx primitiva, instead of migrating in between the split cords, would pass around it to accumulate dorsally. These cells then pass between the two hemicords from dorsal to ventral direction, thus causing the formation of the dorsal spur. The rarity of this condition has precluded any definite proof of these theories.

Demography

The reported cases in literature have been summarized in **Table 6.1**. The occurrence of dorsal spur shows an equal predilection for both males and females (out of the available data). The relatively recent description of this condition might have led to it being missed in most of the large surgical series in literature. A probable estimate might be drawn from the existing data.

Ersahin et al in their analysis of 74 patients with SCM reported 46 girls (62%) and 28 boys (38%).[20] Mahapatra in his study of 300 cases showed that clinical presentation had two peaks, 1 to 3 years of age and also 12 to 16 years of age.[21] Mahapatra and Gupta, in their study of 254 patients with SCM, reported that the patients' ages ranged from 16 days to 35 years (mean age 7.3 years). The mean age of the patients with neurological deficits was 6.66 years, whereas asymptomatic patients presented at a mean age of 6.7 years. As many as 23 of their patients were adults older than 18 years of age, and 60.3% of their patients were female. The common site of SCM was in the lumbar spine, followed by the dorsolumbar area.[20–22] The most common site of dorsal spur is lumbar followed by dorsal, with composite spurs seen in two of the reported cases.

Clinical Features

Of all the reported cases of dorsal spur, half of the patients had no neurological deficits at the time of presentation. Two presented with progressive scoliosis. Of the three patients with neurological deficits in the form of paraparesis, only one had preoperative bowel/bladder involvement (**Table 6.1**). There are no unique clinical features associated with a dorsal spur. The clinical features are similar to other SCM types reported in literature.

These include either *cutaneous* markers such as hypertrichosis, capillary hemangioma, hyper-pigmentation, dimple, scoliosis/kyphoscoliosis, musculocutaneous deformities of the lower limb such as congenital talipes equinovarus (CTEV), or neurological sensorimotor deficits and autonomic disturbances. Weakness and atrophy of limbs, gait disturbances, dysesthetic pain, hypoesthesia, or trophic ulcers may be seen. Bladder and bowel disturbances are also noted.[20–22] Few of the patients might be asymptomatic at presentation.

Table 6.1 Literature review of SCM cases with dorsal spur

Author	Age	Cutaneous stigmata	Symptoms	Location of spur	MRI	Surgery	Postop course	Outcome
Chandra et al[4]	9 years/M	Tuft of hair over lower back	None	L2	Two separate dural tubes, LLTC at L4, HPA	Laminectomy, detethering and removal of spur	Uneventful	Stable at 3-month follow-up
Ersahin[14]	14 months/M	Tuft of hair over lower back	None	L3	Two hemicords in single dural tube, LLTC, HPA	Removal of bony spur and detethering	NA	NA
Akay et al[15]	7 years/F	Tuft of hair over lower back	None	L4	Two hemicords in a single dural tube, LLTC at L4 with HPA	Laminectomy, detethering and removal of bony spur	Uneventful	Stable at 18-month follow-up
	2 years/F	Rigid mass lesion over sacrum	None	S1	Two hemicords in single dural tube, LLTC at coccyx with HPA	Laminectomy, detethering and removal of bony spur	Uneventful	Stable at 3-month follow-up
Sinha et al five cases with dorsal spur[16]	NA	NA	NA	NA	NA	NA	NA	NA
Ailawadhi et al[17]	3 years/F	None	Left lower limb weakness (MRC grade 4/5)	D6, D12, L3 (composite bony spur)	Splitting of the spinal cord at T6, T12 and L3 and the LLTC at L4, with syringomyelia of both hemicords	Laminectomy with removal of bony spurs and detethering	Uneventful	NA

Table 6.1 *Continued*

Table 6.1 (Continued) Literature review of SCM cases with dorsal spur

Author	Age	Cutaneous stigmata	Symptoms	Location of spur	MRI	Surgery	Postop course	Outcome
Prasad et al[18]	2 years/M	None	Kyphoscoliosis, mild paraparesis, urinary and fecal incontinence	D12	SCM from D12 to L1 level (two separate dural tubes), long segment syrinx, low lying conus, HPA	Removal of spur and detethering	Mild worsening of paraparesis	Improvement in motor and autonomic function at 1-year follow-up
	2½ years/F	None	Progressive paraparesis (MRC grade 4/5)	L3	L1–L3 split cord, low-lying conus at L5, HPA	Removal of spur and detethering	Marked paraparesis (MRC Grade 2/5)	Improvement in motor function to preop status at 1-year follow-up
	6 months/M	Tuft of hair over lower back	None	L4	SCM from L2–L5 level, low lying conus at S1	Removal of spur and detethering	Uneventful	Stable at 14-month follow-up
	3 years/F	Pigmented patch over lower back	Kyphoscoliosis	D4	SCM from D4–D6	Removal of spur	Uneventful	Stable at 1-year follow-up
Garg et al[19]	16 months/M	None	Scoliosis	D11–L3 (complete at D11, partial Y-shaped below that)	Two hemicords with syrinx in separate dural sheaths, LLTC at L4	Laminectomy with removal of bony spur and detethering	Uneventful	NA

Abbreviations: HPA, hypertrophied posterior arch; LLTC, low-lying tethered cord; MRC, medical research council; SCM, split cord malformation.

Imaging Studies

Imaging forms the mainstay of diagnosis of a dorsal spur. Recent advances in the form of high-resolution MRI can accurately define the location, extent, orientation, and attachments of the midline septum (**Fig. 6.1** and **Fig. 6.2**). Whole spine MRI should be performed in all suspected patients to find out the number of involved segments, any concurrent sites of defects, and other associated anomalies like lipoma, thick filum, dermoid and epidermoid tumors, neurenteric cyst or dermal sinus. Whole spine MRI is especially important to detect cases of composite spurs. The cervical spine should be evaluated to rule out any associated Chiari malformation and craniovertebral junction anomalies. A CT scan can be helpful to define the exact bony extent of the spur. Dorsal spur starts at the ventral surface of the posterior elements and is partial in nature, that is, it does not go all the way up to the vertebral body with which it might have a fibrocartilaginous attachment. Further, CT scan helps in demonstration of HPA, with which half the reported cases of dorsal spur are associated with.

Treatment

Surgical excision of the spur along with detethering of the cord is the treatment of choice.[4,18] Some of the surgical steps involved vary when compared to surgery for the commonly described variants of SCM. Spinal laminae should never be removed en bloc when dealing with a dorsal spur.[4,18] This is due to the

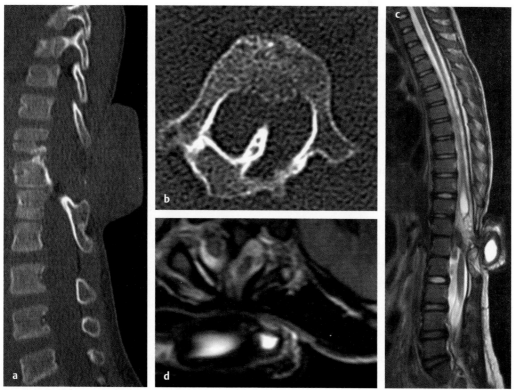

Fig. 6.1 (a–d) CT and MRI showing SCM type I with dorsoventral spur with associated meningocele. Note the hypertrophied posterior arch (HPA) in the axial CT image.

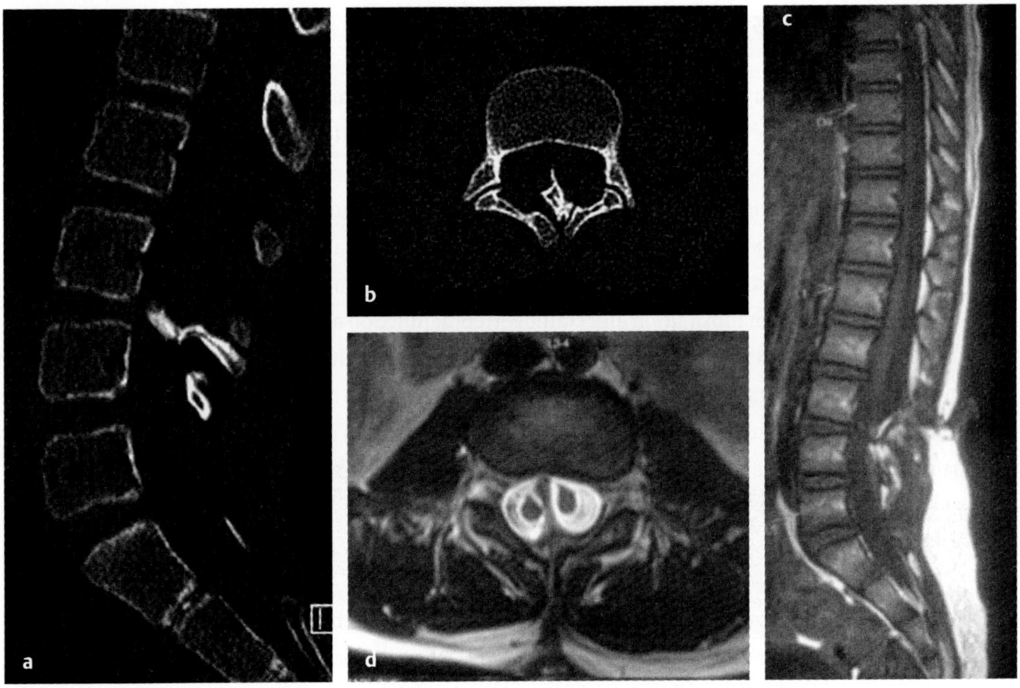

Fig. 6.2 (a–d) Another case of SCM type I with CT and MRI cuts showing a dorsoventral spur.

potential risk of damaging the spinal cord by the ventral end of the spur, which is not attached to the vertebral body. Thus, the overlying lamina should be drilled in an unhurried manner. The dorsal end of the spur should be isolated and cautiously drilled off. The thinned-out portion of the spur may be removed with microronguers. Once the dorsal spur has been dealt with, the rest of the surgery proceeds in a manner similar to the repair of other SCMs.[4,18] The dura is opened in the conventional fashion and a sufficient length is mobilized to allow for watertight dural closure. After duraplasty, the wound is closed in layers.

Patient Outcome

There are very limited cases available in literature to draw any definite conclusions. By all accounts, a careful surgical dissection and detethering has a favorable outcome (**Table 6.1**). Among the asymptomatic patients with a dorsal spur, none developed fresh neurological deficit. One patient showed worsening of power in the immediate postoperative period, which had improved to preoperative status at 1-year follow-up. Two patients with preoperative deficits showed improvement on follow-up.

Conclusion

Dorsally situated bony spur is an extremely rare entity. MRI complemented with a CT scan is the diagnostic modality of choice. A HPA should raise suspicion of an underlying dorsal spur. Special care must be taken during its surgical excision, which includes cautious drilling of the bony spur. Doing so can lead to a good outcome for the patient.

References

1. Pang D, Dias MS, Ahab-Barmada M. Split cord malformation: Part I: A unified theory of embryogenesis for double spinal cord malformations. Neurosurgery 1992;31(3):451–480

2. Pang D. Split cord malformations. In: Pang D, ed. Disorders of the Pediatric Spine. New York: Raven Press; 1995:203–52

3. Pang D. Split cord malformation: Part II: Clinical syndrome. Neurosurgery 1992;31(3):481–500

4. Chandra PS, Kamal R, Mahapatra AK. An unusual case of dorsally situated bony spur in a lumbar split cord malformation. Pediatr Neurosurg 1999;31(1):49–52

5. Ollivier C. Traité des Maladies de la Moelle Épinière. Paris: Mequignon-Marvis; 1837

6. Bruce A, M'Donald S, Pirie JH. A second case of partial doubling of the spinal cord. Rev Neurol Psychiatry. 1906;4:6–19

7. Feller A, Sternberg H. Zur Kenntnis der Fehlbildungen der Wirbelsäule: I. Die Wirbelkörperspalte und ihre formale Genese. Virchows Arch Am 1929;272:613–640

8. Gardner WJ. Myelocele: rupture of the neural tube? Clin Neurosurg 1968;15:57–79

9. Lichtenstein BW. "Spinal dysraphism"—Spina bifida and myelodysplasia. Arch Neurol Psychiatry 1929;44:792–810

10. Hendrick EB. On diastematomyelia. Prog Neurol Surg 1971;4:277–288

11. Cohen J, Sledge CB. Diastematomyelia. An embryological interpretation with report of a case. Am J Dis Child 1960;100:257–263

12. Müller F, O'Rahilly R. The development of the human brain, the closure of the caudal neuropore, and the beginning of secondary neurulation at stage 12. Anat Embryol (Berl) 1987;176(4):413–430

13. Beardmore HE, Wiglesworth FW. Vertebral anomalies and alimentary duplications; clinical and embryological aspects. Pediatr Clin North Am 1958;5:457–474

14. Erşahin Y. An unusual split cord malformation. Pediatr Neurosurg 2000;32(2):109

15. Akay KM, Izci Y, Baysefer A. Dorsal bony septum: a split cord malformation variant. Pediatr Neurosurg 2002;36(5):225–228

16. Sinha S, Agarwal D, Mahapatra AK. Split cord malformations: an experience of 203 cases. Childs Nerv Syst 2006;22(1):3–7

17. Ailawadhi P, Mahapatra AK. An unusual case of spinal dysraphism with four splits including three posterior spurs. Pediatr Neurosurg 2011;47(5):372–375

18. Prasad GL, Borkar SA, Satyarthee GD, Mahapatra AK. Split cord malformation with dorsally located bony spur: Report of four cases and review of literature. J Pediatr Neurosci 2012;7(3):167–170

19. Garg K, Tandon V, Mahapatra AK. A unique case of split cord malformation type 1 with three different types of bony spurs. Asian J Neurosurg 2017;12(2):305–308

20. Erşahin Y, Mutluer S, Kocaman S, Demirtaş E. Split spinal cord malformations in children. J Neurosurg 1998;88(1):57–65

21. Mahapatra AK. Split cord malformation—A study of 300 cases at AIIMS 1990–2006. J Pediatr Neurosci 2011;6(Suppl 1):S41–S45

22. Mahapatra AK, Gupta DK. Split cord malformations: a clinical study of 254 patients and a proposal for a new clinical-imaging classification. J Neurosurg 2005; 103(6, Suppl):531–536

4. ...

5. Weights Politics Committees, Department of Health, ... childhood obesity in Britain, Plan/Strategy 1999/08 [117–127].

6. Hedayati S ... care coordination ... a novel ... AIIMS 1999–2006, Ped et Senan 98, 1 (suppl.) 1504 (1–5).

7. Vedprakash AK, Gupta R K. ... cost multi/multivariate ... in children ... deprivation and implications for a new clinical imaging ... short term, Pediatrica 2006, IJRA-Suppl 331–338.

CHAPTER 7

Cervical Split Cord Malformations

Sachin A. Borkar, Ravi Sreenivasan, and Ashok K. Mahapatra

Table of Contents

- Introduction 63

- Embryology 63

- Pathophysiology of Symptoms 64

- Epidemiology 64

- Clinical Symptoms 72

- Investigations 72

- Indications for Surgery 73

- Surgical Technique 73

- Results of Surgery 74

- Complications 74

- Summary... 75

Cervical Split Cord Malformations

Sachin A. Borkar, Ravi Sreenivasan, and Ashok K. Mahapatra

Introduction

The term "diastematomyelia" was coined by Ollivier from Greek *diastema–* cleft and *melos–* medulla.[1,2] It describes a congenital cleft, or splitting of the spinal cord, each division of which may be invested in a distinct arachnoid sheath under a common dura or may have separate dural sheaths.[2,3] Von Recklinghausen coined the term *diplomyelia* to describe a completely formed spinal cord situated anteriorly or posteriorly to the native cord.[4] Herren and Edwards defined the term *diplomyelia* (Greek *dipulo–* double) to include any complete duplication of a spinal cord segment.[5] Although better antenatal screening and care have resulted in a worldwide declining trend in the incidence of neural tube defects overall, the widespread availability of MRI and active surveillance of scoliosis patients being referred for treatment have resulted in this condition being increasingly reported from the Indian subcontinent.[6]

Embryology

In 1892, Hertwig was the first to experimentally produce this malformation in frogs by delaying the fertilization of the ovum. Hamby (1936) is credited as the first surgeon to have operated on a living patient with diastematomyelia.[7]

Pang et al suggested the phrase "split cord malformations" (SCM) to describe the entire gamut of anomalies associated.[8] According to Pang,[8] the embryological error that leads to a SCM is the formation of an abnormal fistulous tract through the midline embryonic disc. This fistula preserves a communication between the yolk sac and the amnion, which makes a persistent contact between the ectoderm and endoderm feasible. This leads to localized splitting of the notochord and the overlying neural plate. The enveloping pluripotent mesenchymal tissue condenses around the fistulous tract to form an endomesenchymal tract that divides the notochord and forces each overlying half to neurulate against its own hemicord.

The basic anomaly thus comprises two heminotochords and two hemineural plates separated by a midline fistulous tract containing ectoderm, endoderm, and mesenchyme. Further evolution of this anomaly into final malformation depends on the ability of the hemicords and heminotochords to heal around the fistula, the fate of the three germinal elements within this fistula, the variable extent and duration to which this fistula persists, as well as the interaction between the heminotochord and the hemineural plates during neurulation.

Pang et al classified SCMs into types I and II.

- Type I SCM: It is characterized by two hemicords, each contained within its own dural sac, and separated by an osseocartilagenous septum.

- Type II SCM: It is characterized by two hemicords in the same dural sac, separated by a fibrous septum

Mahapatra and Gupta further state that the midline bone most likely originates from these very precursor meninges, which also give rise to the dural tubes. After the formation of the dural tube, the precursor meninx on the side of the median dura which faces each hemicord forms a complete arachnoid tube, and the precursor meninx on the side facing the midline forms the bony spur. The extent of the remnants of the endomesenchymal fistula and the subsequent interaction of precursor meninges with the residual fistula determines the position of spur. This is probably genetically controlled.[9] Many cases of cervical SCM are associated with Klippel–Feil (KF) syndrome and other disorders of vertebral fusion and segmentation. The influences of homeobox genes Pax-1 and Hox are being investigated but the relationship between the genes affecting spinal cord division and primary segmentation as yet remains unknown.[10] Chandra et al[11] postulated two mechanisms for the occurrence of a dorsal spur, a rare variant: (1) passage of an abnormal cell cluster dorsally with subsequent loss of contact with the ventrally situated cell cluster and (2) migration of cells around the hemicords and formation of passage between them in a dorsoventral direction.

Pathophysiology of Symptoms

■ Mechanical Factors

The osseous/fibrous-cartilaginous septum tethers the spinal cord and impedes its normal ascent with growth of the skeleton, leading to tethering of the cord. The plasticity of the nervous system allows for small children to remain asymptomatic for long. However, with growth spurt, this plasticity is also rendered ineffective and patients become symptomatic. This tethered cord that is not normally floating in cerebrospinal fluid (CSF) space is further insulted by coexisting spinal stenosis and deformity.[12–14]

■ Vascular Factors

An asymmetrical distribution of blood supply to the hemicords and compression of the anterior spinal artery or veins leads to ischemic disturbances which, in turn, leads to symptoms.[15,16] Yamada et al demonstrated the effect of traction on vascular supply to the spinal cord of a cat using spectroscopy.[17]

■ Anatomical Factors

Hypoplasia of one or both of the hemicords may give rise to any of the symptoms encountered.[8]

Epidemiology

Till 1972, most of the 11 cases described were diagnoses made at autopsy, with the earliest report by Fischer et al in 1889.[18] James et al (1972) were the first to document the clinical picture in a 56-year-old woman with quadriplegia.[18] Whittle et al (1983) were one of the first authors to document the successful surgical outcome of spur excision and repair in a 2-year-old girl with KF syndrome who presented with posttraumatic paraparesis.[19] There have been sporadic reports every year or two since then, with the largest series reported by Mahapatra et al[6,9] (nine cases, 2011). Previously, David et al[10] (seven cases, 1996) and Ulmer et al[20] (five cases, 1993) had reported the presence of cervical SCM in patients of KF syndrome. To date, less than 75 cases of cervical SCMs (**Fig. 7.1**) have been reported in worldwide literature (**Table 7.1**).

The age of presentation has ranged from the newborn to as late as 56 years of age, with approximately 50% cases (30 cases) presenting before the age of 10.[6,9,18,19,21–28] As many as 23 cases have been described in adults over the age of 18.[10,14,18,20,29–38] A female preponderance is evident (M:F | 2:5). The reason for this distribution remains as yet unexplained.

Although reported from all over the world, few reports have come from Japan[32,34] and the African nations, whereas large series have emanated from India[6,9,39] and Turkey.[37,40] Underdiagnosis and underreporting could be one reason. There could be ethnic or environmental factors that are still to be unearthed.

The reports of cervical SCM have been too sporadic to discern a familial inheritance pattern.

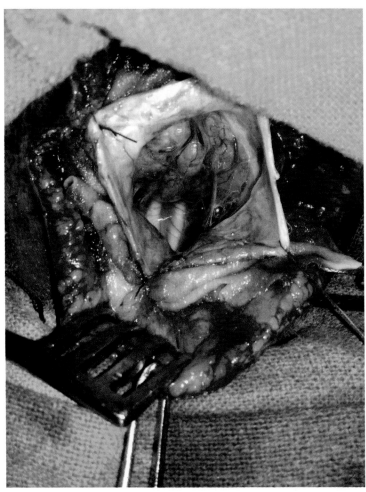

Fig. 7.1 Intraoperative picture showing a high cervical split cord malformation. Note the cerebellum in upper part of the picture. (Reproduced with permission from Sreenivasan R, Sharma R, Borkar SA, et al. Cervical split cord malformations: a systematic review. Neurol India 2020;68:994–1002.)

Table 7.1 71 documented cases of cervical SCM reported in literature from 1889 to 2016

S. No.	Author	Age/Sex	Level	Associated anomalies	Symptoms	Treatment	Outcome	Cervical cases	Total cases	Year
1	Fischer[18]	Newborn	Upper Cervical	Spina bifida, MMC, clubfoot	NR, autopsy diagnosis	-	Died	1	1	1889
2	Ammon[18]	-	Cervical and upper thoracic	Spina bifida	NR, autopsy diagnosis	-	Died	1	1	1906
3	Avery[18]	35 d/F	C1-T4	Sprengel shoulder, KF syndrome, torticollis, strabismus, wide palpebral fissure	NR, autopsy diagnosis	-	Died	1	1	1936
4	Walker[18]	4/F	C6	Spina bifida occulta	Traumatic quadri-paresis with polio	-	Died	1	1	1944
5	Gunderson[41]	11/M	Upper cervical	KF syndrome, arachnodactyly, webbed neck, low set ears	NR, autopsy diagnosis	On treatment for pneumonia	Died	1	1	1968
6	Mackenzie[18]	Infants	Last two cervical segments	Chiari type 2	NR, autopsy diagnosis	-	Died	6	6	1971
7	James[18]	56/F	C4-C5	NR	Quadriplegia	Refused surgery	NR	1	1	1972
8	Giordano[42]	11/M	C1	None	Quadriparesis	NR	NR	1	1	1982
9	Naidich[21]	3/F	C7-T1	Chiari type 2	NR	-	NR	1	1	1983
10	Whittle[19]	2/F	C6-C7	KF, webbed neck	Posttrauma paraparesis	Laminectomy and excision	Complete recovery	1	1	1983

Table 7.1 Continued

Table 7.1 (Continued) 71 documented cases of cervical SCM reported in literature from 1889 to 2016

S. No.	Author	Age/Sex	Level	Associated anomalies	Symptoms	Treatment	Outcome	Cervical cases	Total cases	Year
11	Beyerl[29]	34/F	C2-C3	4 café au lait spots	Quadriparesis with bowel and bladder involvement following assault	Laminectomy and excision	Improved slowly	1	1	1985
12	Anand[30] Kuchner[31]	20/F	C5-C6	Bifid C6 arch, cervical rib, 5 × 7 cm nevus over back	Left hemiparesis following trauma	Laminectomy and excision	Complete motor recovery	1	1	1985
13	Levine[43]	14/F	Inferior cervical	KF syndrome, thoracolumbar scoliosis	Mild sensory paresis in lower limbs	Conservative	NR	1	1	1985
14	Simpson[18]	19/M	C6-C7	Webbed neck, blunt facies, ptosis, short thick arms, multiple hernias, gynecomastia, urethral stricture	Traumatic quadriparesis	Laminectomy and excision	Improved motor power	1	1	1986
15	Okada[32]	19/M	C3-C5	Cervical kyphosis	Right upper limb paresthesias and muscle wasting	Conservative	Stable course	1	1	1986
16	Wolf[14]	27/M	C2-C4	KF syndrome, short neck, decreased neck motion	Quadriparesis, sensory loss in both lower limbs, impotence, and incontinence	Laminectomy and excision	Slow improvement with persistent spasticity	1	1	1987
17	Nakamura[33]	19/M 24/F	C3-C6 C4-T1	-	Right upper limb monoparesis, right upper limb monoparesis	-	-	2	2	1989

Table 7.1 Continued

Table 7.1 (Continued) 71 documented cases of cervical SCM reported in literature from 1889 to 2016

S. No.	Author	Age/Sex	Level	Associated anomalies	Symptoms	Treatment	Outcome	Cervical cases	Total cases	Year
18	Ohwada[34]	29/M	C6-C7	None	Progressive paraparesis, urinary incontinence	Laminectomy and excision	Improved motor power and incontinence	1	1	1989
19	Pfeifer[23] Herman[22]	Newborn/F	Basicranium to T1	Optic nerve coloboma, Dandy–Walker cyst, occipital meningocele, malformed posterior fossa structures with two cords coming out of foramen magnum	Respiratory failure at birth, autopsy diagnosis	-	Died at 14 days	1	1	1990 1991
20	Rawanduzy[35]	33/F	C6	None	Posttraumatic right upper limb weakness and paresthesias	ACDF with spur excision	Complete recovery	1	1	1991
21	Pang[8]	5 children 1 adult (C7)	C4 (2 cases) C7 (4 cases)	5/6 had conus at L1 and 1/6 had a conus tethered by terminal lipoma at L2. One child with type II SCM had complete malrotation of midgut with partial obstruction of duodenum	4/6 patients had progressive neural deficits, paresthesiae of upper limbs and clumsiness with/without leg spasticity	Laminectomy and excision of spur	Improved	6	41	1992

Table 7.1 Continued

Table 7.1 (Continued) 71 documented cases of cervical SCM reported in literature from 1889 to 2016

S. No.	Author	Age/Sex	Level	Associated anomalies	Symptoms	Treatment	Outcome	Cervical cases	Total cases	Year
22	Ulmer[20]	10/M 15/F 24/F 29/F 38/M	C1-3 C5-T1 C2-7 C1-3 C1-2	KF syndrome	KF syndrome, neck pain, Radiculopathy dystonia, weakness	NR	NR	5	24 KF	1993
23	Birch[36]	48/F	High cervical	Congenital mirror movement	-	-	-	1	1	1996
24	David[10]	54/F 11/F 13/F 24/F 10/F 36/F 35/F	C0-C3 C1-C7 C1-C3 C0-C3 C1-C3 C0-C3 C1-C3	KF syndrome, meningocele	KF syndrome, neck pain, radiculopathy	Conservative (5) Excision and shunt (1) OC3 fusion (1)	Stable	7	7 KF	1996
25	Jaeger[44]	16/F	C1 to Lumbar spine	Lumbar MMC with hydrocephalus at birth, ureterostomy	Complete paraplegia with gradual onset progressive weakness of upper limbs	Laminectomy, detethering and shunting of syringes into subcutaneous reservoir	Slow improvement in upper limbs	1	1	1996
26	Androni kou[24]	8/M	-	KF	-	-	-	1	1 KF	2001
27	Balci[26]	2/F	C0-C7	Wildervanck syndrome	Mental retardation, nystagmus, hearing loss	-	-	1	1	2002

Table 7.1 Continued

Table 7.1 *(Continued)* 71 documented cases of cervical SCM reported in literature from 1889 to 2016

S. No.	Author	Age/Sex	Level	Associated anomalies	Symptoms	Treatment	Outcome	Cervical cases	Total cases	Year
28	Myles[26]	1/F	C7-T1	Tethered cord at T1, meningocele C6-7	Mental retardation, anesthesia in upper limbs, floppy child, incontinence	Laminectomy and excision	Persistent incontinence, persistent hypoesthesia, improved hand function	1	1	2002
29	Korinth[25,28]	2/M	C4-C5	Hypertrichosis at C7T1, scoliosis, intradural epidermoid cyst	Normal neurology, Scoliosis	Laminectomy and excision	Normal neurology	1	1	2004
30	Mahapatra[6,9]	7.3 mean M:F (2:3)	Cervical and cervicodorsal	Varied	Varied	Laminotomy and excision	Varied 50% cases improved	9 (7 cervical + 2 cervicodorsal)	254 300	2005 2011
31	Rustamzadeh[27]	1	Basicranial to C1	Asymmetrical face, bilateral internal foot rotation	General hypotonia, hemifacial microsomia, and developmental delay	Complete resection of the cutaneous sinus tract and the lipoma within the arachnoid cyst wall	Slow improvement of motor power	1	1	2006
32	Ozturk[37]	30.1 mean M:F (9:14)	Cervical and cervicodorsal	Varied	Varied	-	-	3	23	2008
33	Andro[45]	11/M	C7T1	Short neck, splitting of vertebral bodies from C3-T7	Normal neurology	Conservative	Stable Normal neurology	1	1	2009

Table 7.1 Continued

Table 7.1 (Continued) 71 documented cases of cervical SCM reported in literature from 1889 to 2016

S. No.	Author	Age/Sex	Level	Associated anomalies	Symptoms	Treatment	Outcome	Cervical cases	Total cases	Year
34	Orakdogen[40]	9/F	C6-7	Mass lesion at C6-7 (MMC)	Normal neurology	Laminectomy + excision and repair	Normal neurology	1 SCM + MMC rest MMC	7	2009
35	Huang[28]	18 m /F	C5-6	Cervical MMC	Normal neurology	Resection, detethering	Normal neurology	1	10	2010
36	Borkar[39]	-	-	Hypertrichosis	-	Laminectomy + excision	50% improved	3	53	2012
37	Oyar[38]	18/F	Basicranium to C2	Occipitocervical mass	Normal neurology	Refused surgery	Stable	1	1	2012
38	Maloney[46]	7 days/F	Basicranium to C2	Left-sided torticollis left vocal cord paresis,	Apneic episodes, progressive lethargy, difficulty feeding, and noisy breathing during sleep	Suboccipital craniectomy, cord untethering, bovine duraplasty	Normal growth with persistent torticollis	1	1	2016

Abbreviations: ACDF, anterior cervical discectomy and fusion; KF, Klippel-Feil syndrome; MMC: meningomyelocele; NR: not reported; OC: occipitocervical; SCM: split cord malformation.

Clinical Symptoms

- Normal neurology (seen in as many as 15% cases).[25,28,38,40,43,45]
- Overwhelming majority (>50%) show some degree of neural deficits.
- Neck pain.
- Torticollis.
- Radiculopathies.
- Neurotrophic ulcer: A peculiar characteristic that has often led to the diagnosis is the self-mutilation of fingers due to sucking and biting the anesthetic limb.[47]
- Neurotrophic joints.
- Clubfoot deformities and pes cavus.
- Spinal deformities: kyphosis, scoliosis, kyphoscoliosis.
- Wasting of lower limbs.
- Gait disturbances: varying degrees of spasticity, clumsiness, ataxia (if syringobulbia is present).
- Varying level of motor deficits: from normal power to frank quadriplegia. Even thoracic myelopathy has been the initial presenting feature.[34] Hemiplegia following trivial trauma has also been reported.[30] In fact, significant neural deficits disproportionate to the trivial trauma in adults has often led to the finding of SCMs in an otherwise normal adult.[35]
- Varying severity of bladder and bowel incontinence.
- Cutaneous stigmata including hypertrichosis, naevi, dimples, dermal sinus, lipomatous swellings (seen in as many as 60% cases).[6]
- Other neural tube defects like meningocele and meningomyelocele may coexist.
- Associated features of KF syndrome including low-lying hairline with limitation of neck movements, Sprengel shoulder (high riding scapula with an omovertebral bar), pterygium colli (webbed neck), symmetrical/mirror movements of the upper limbs.

Investigations

■ Antenatal Diagnosis

There are isolated case reports in literature mentioning the use of antenatal sonogram and MRI for establishing the diagnosis.[48–52] However, routine antenatal sonogram (level 2 scan) should be routinely utilized to look for any marker of associated neural tube defects that may lead to the diagnosis of a SCM.

■ Postnatal Diagnosis

- Ultrasonogram: screening tool of choice for detection of suspected SCM and is superior to a plain radiograph in newborns.
- MRI: A screening MRI covering the whole spine is mandatory in all suspected cases to detect occult multisite dysraphisms.[6,9] MRI is the definitive investigation of choice and can delineate the exact morphology of the cord and anomalies such as:
  ◇ Hemicords.

◇ Syrinx.

◇ Intradural malformations:

- Fatty filum.

- Teratomas/dermoids.

- Lipomas.

- Cysts.

- CT scan should be performed for highlighting the bony elements of the anomaly and their relationship with the cord, especially when associated with scoliosis or kyphosis. Conversely, all patients planned for spinal deformity correction should be screened for occult or overt spinal dysraphism before proceeding for surgery.

■ Role of Urodynamics

Perez et al[53] stated that all patients with SCM should undergo a urodynamic evaluation prior to surgical intervention. It helps in prognosticating postoperative outcome as well. As much as 60 to 75% patients with SCM have subtle or overt urinary tract dysfunction, with the most common complaint being urge incontinence.[53,54] They usually tend to stabilize or improve after surgery.

Indications for Surgery

The need for surgery in an asymptomatic patient is a question that has been debated for long. The treatment of intraspinal anomalies prior to deformity correction results in better outcomes is a fact endorsed by most orthopedists and neurosurgeons who operate on spinal deformities.[55,56]

David et al reserved surgery for only those with overt spinal instability and progressive neural deficit.[10] Only 1/7 cases in their series were operated. Zuccaro states that majority of asymptomatic patients in their series were not operated and did well at 7-year follow-up.[57] However, Matson et al,[58] Mahapatra et al,[6] and Proctor et al[54] have all suggested that the aim of the surgery should be prophylactic rather than curative and as such, should be offered to asymptomatic patients as well.

Surgery often leads to healing of trophic ulcers as well.[9] Surgery is definitely indicated in all patients who present with associated anomalies like dermal sinus, dermoids, teratomas, and cysts that can by themselves lead to complications if not treated appropriately.

Surgical Technique

Patients are operated in a prone position. Intraoperative neurophysiological monitoring (IONM) by means of motor-evoked potentials (MEP) and somatosensory-evoked potentials (SSEP) is the current standard of care but depends on the availability of trained personnel and equipment. Intraoperative monitoring can give the surgeon greater confidence while dissecting and manipulating around the cord by guiding him or her to stop dissection till the reduced amplitude of evoked potentials returns to baseline levels. The use of intraoperative image intensifier/X-ray/navigation is needed to correctly localize the site of the lesion, as cutaneous stigmata can be segments away from the actual lesion.

A laminotomy or laminectomy with a high-speed drill/burr is done and a Kerrison's punch (or a diamond drill) can be used to nibble out the spur completely before proceeding with detethering as needed.[9] A laminoplasty is indicated for large segment disease to prevent postlaminectomy kyphosis. Alternatively, pedicle screw fixation can be combined with the procedure, especially if deformity correction is done in the same sitting. The dural sleeve of the spur must be completely removed, as there have been reports of new spurs arising from reossification along the remnant sleeve.[59-61] Division of the filum detethers the cord.[6] This is done by a small sacral laminotomy in cases of cervical SCM.

For dorsally located spurs, a laminoplasty should never be performed for fear of causing cord damage.[62] A laminectomy one level above and one below the level of the spur is done. The spur is removed gradually in a dorsal to ventral direction, and the dura is opened with a gentle curve encircling the spur. The durotomy is extended about two levels cephalad and caudad to the level of the lesion, so that there remains sufficient dura for watertight closure. The bony spur is thinned out with a high-speed drill and the shell remaining is removed with microrongeurs. Watertight dural closure is done with 5-0 vicryl or nylon. The rest of the wound is closed in layers.

Results of Surgery

Multiple surgeons have reported gratifying results of surgery, with dramatic improvement in neurology to complete recovery of symptoms reported.[6,18,19,25,28,29,31,34,35,40] Persistent neural deficits or incomplete recovery are also reported in some cases with severe preoperative deficits.[14,27,39,47] Retethering may occur in 7 to 10% patients over a period of 5 years due to reossification of spur along any remnant dural sleeve.[59-61] Mahapatra reported that none of the patients undergoing prophylactic surgery had postoperative neurological deterioration.[6]

Complications

Overall, the complications of SCM surgery are low.

Perioperative complications are related to distorted anatomy and difficulties with hemostasis and water-tight dura closure.

Mahapatra and Gupta subclassified type I SCM into four types, based on the position of the bony spur causing the split.[9]

1. Type Ia: The bone spur lays in the center of the split, with an equally duplicated cord above and below the spur.
2. Type Ib: The bone spur is situated at the superior pole, with no space above it, and a large duplicated cord lower down.
3. Type Ic: The bone spur is situated on the lower pole, with a large duplicated cord above.
4. Type Id: The bone spur is straddling the bifurcation of the spinal cord, with no space above or below the spur.

The risk of inflicting trauma to the hemicords is highest in Type 1d, as four out of six patients with type Id anomalies in their series had postoperative deterioration.[9] Postoperative urinary retention, arachnoiditis, and infections are also reported complications which are managed conservatively.[9,63]

Summary

- Cervical SCM is, fortunately, an exceptionally rare condition, with less than 75 cases documented in literature.

- MRI remains the investigation of choice for diagnosis, planning treatment, and follow-up.

- The debate regarding prophylactic surgery in asymptomatic individuals continues. However, the authors advocate prophylactic surgery in all asymptomatic individuals to preclude severe neurological deficit following trivial trauma in future.

- The results of surgery in asymptomatic individuals are excellent while those in symptomatic individuals are fairly good as well.

- Routine screening for cord anomalies should be done for all cases undergoing orthopedic deformity correction surgeries to prevent inadvertent perioperative catastrophes.

References

1. Ollivier C. Traité des Maladies de la Moelle Épinière., 3rd ed. Paris: Méquignon Marvis; 1837
2. Cohen J, Sledge CB. Diastematomyelia. An embryological interpretation with report of a case. Am J Dis Child 1960;100:257–263
3. Hertwig O. Urmund und Spina Bifida. Arch Mikr Anat 1892;39:353–503
4. Von Recklinghausen F. Untersuchungen über die spina bifida. Virchows Arch Path Anat 1886;105:243–330
5. Herren RY, Edwards JE. Diplomyelia (duplication of the spinal cord). Arch Path 1940;30:1203–1214
6. Mahapatra AK. Split cord malformation—a study of 300 cases at AIIMS 1990-2006. J Pediatr Neurosci 2011;6(Suppl 1):S41–S45
7. Hamby W. Pilonidal cyst, spina bifida occulta abd bifid spinal cord. Report of a case with review of the literature. Arch Pathol (Chic) 1936;21:831–838
8. Pang D, Dias MS, Ahab-Barmada M. Split cord malformation: Part I: A unified theory of embryogenesis for double spinal cord malformations. Neurosurgery 1992;31(3):451–480
9. Mahapatra AK, Gupta DK. Split cord malformations: a clinical study of 254 patients and a proposal for a new clinical-imaging classification. J Neurosurg 2005; 103(6, Suppl):531–536
10. David KM, Copp AJ, Stevens JM, Hayward RD, Crockard HA. Split cervical spinal cord with Klippel-Feil syndrome: seven cases. Brain 1996;119(Pt 6):1859–1872
11. Chandra PS, Kamal R, Mahapatra AK. An unusual case of dorsally situated bony spur in a lumbar split cord malformation. Pediatr Neurosurg 1999;31(1):49–52
12. Pang D, Wilberger JE Jr. Tethered cord syndrome in adults. J Neurosurg 1982;57(1):32–47
13. Pang D. Ventral tethering in split cord malformation. Neurosurg Focus 2001;10(1):e6
14. Wolf AL, Tubman DE, Seljeskog EL. Diastematomyelia of the cervical spinal cord with tethering in an adult. Neurosurgery 1987;21(1):94–98
15. Vandresse JH, Cornelis G. Diastematomyelia: report of eight observations. Neuroradiology 1975;10(2):87–93
16. Hülser PJ, Schroth G, Petersen D. Magnetic resonance and CT imaging of diastematomyelia. Eur Arch Psychiatry Neurol Sci 1985;235(2):107–109
17. Yamada S, Zinke DE, Sanders D. Pathophysiology of "tethered cord syndrome". J Neurosurg 1981;54(4):494–503
18. Simpson RK Jr, Rose JE. Cervical diastematomyelia. Report of a case and review of a rare congenital anomaly. Arch Neurol 1987;44(3):331–335

19. Whittle IR, Besser M. Congenital neural abnormalities presenting with mirror movements in a patient with Klippel-Feil syndrome. Case report. J Neurosurg 1983;59(5):891–894

20. Ulmer JL, Elster AD, Ginsberg LE, Williams DW III. Klippel-Feil syndrome: CT and MR of acquired and congenital abnormalities of cervical spine and cord. J Comput Assist Tomogr 1993;17(2):215–224

21. Naidich TP, McLone DG, Fulling KH. The Chiari II malformation: Part IV. The hindbrain deformity. Neuroradiology 1983;25(4):179–197

22. Herman TE, Siegel MJ. Cervical and basicranial diastematomyelia. AJR Am J Roentgenol 1990;154(4):806–808

23. Pfeifer JD. Basicranial diastematomyelia: a case report. Clin Neuropathol 1991;10(5):232–236

24. Andronikou S, Fieggeru AG. Klippel-Feil syndrome with cervical diastematomyelia in an 8-year-old boy. Pediatr Radiol 2001;31(9):636

25. Korinth MC, Kapser A, Nolte K, Gilsbach JM. Cervical diastematomyelia associated with an intradural epidermoid cyst between the hemicords and multiple vertebral body anomalies. Pediatr Neurosurg 2004;40(5):253–256

26. Balci S, Oguz KK, Firat MM, Boduroglu K. Cervical diastematomyelia in cervico-oculo-acoustic (Wildervanck) syndrome: MRI findings. Clin Dysmorphol 2002;11(2):125–128

27. Rustamzadeh E, Graupman PC, Lam CH. Basicranial diplomyelia: an extension of the split cord malformation theory. Case report. J Neurosurg 2006; 104(5, Suppl):362–365

28. Huang SL, Shi W, Zhang LG. Characteristics and surgery of cervical myelomeningocele. Childs Nerv Syst 2010;26(1):87–91

29. Beyerl BD, Ojemann RG, Davis KR, Hedley-Whyte ET, Mayberg MR. Cervical diastematomyelia presenting in adulthood. Case report. J Neurosurg 1985;62(3):449–453

30. Anand AK, Kuchner E, James R. Cervical diastematomyelia: uncommon presentation of a rare congenital disorder. Comput Radiol 1985;9(1):45–49

31. Kuchner EF, Anand AK, Kaufman BM. Cervical diastematomyelia: a case report with operative management. Neurosurgery 1985;16(4):538–542

32. Okada K, Fuji T, Yonenobu K, Ono K. Cervical diastematomyelia with a stable neurological deficit. Report of a case. J Bone Joint Surg Am 1986;68(6):934–937

33. Nakamura Y, Soga F, Takahashi M, Tarui S, Yamashita K. [Two patients with cervical diastematomyelia]. Rinsho Shinkeigaku 1989;29(3):371–375

34. Ohwada T, Okada K, Hayashi H. Thoracic myelopathy caused by cervicothoracic diastematomyelia. A case report. J Bone Joint Surg Am 1989;71(2):296–299

35. Rawanduzy A, Murali R. Cervical spine diastematomyelia in adulthood. Neurosurgery 1991;28(3):459–461

36. Birch BD, McCormick PC. High cervical split cord malformation and neurenteric cyst associated with congenital mirror movements: case report. Neurosurgery 1996;38(4):813–815, discussion 815–816

37. Ozturk E, Sonmez G, Mutlu H, et al. Split-cord malformation and accompanying anomalies. J Neuroradiol 2008;35(3):150–156

38. Oyar O, Ismailoglu O, Albayrak B. Coexistence of occipital and infratorcular meningocele with cervical split cord anomaly. Singapore Med J 2012;53(7):e145–e147

39. Borkar SA, Mahapatra AK. Split cord malformations: a two years experience at AIIMS. Asian J Neurosurg 2012;7(2):56–60

40. Orakdogen M, Turk CC, Ersahin M, Biber N, Berkman Z. Spinal dysraphisms of the cervicothoracic region in childhood. Turk Neurosurg 2009;19(4):400–405

41. Gunderson CH, Solitare GB. Mirror movements in patients with the Klippel-Feil syndrome. Neuropathologic observations. Arch Neurol 1968;18(6):675–679

42. Giordano GB, Davidovits P, Cerisoli M, Giulioni M. Cervical diplomyelia revealed by computed tomography (CT). Neuropediatrics 1982;13(2):93–94

43. Levine RS, Geremia GK, McNeill TW. CT demonstration of cervical diastematomyelia. J Comput Assist Tomogr 1985;9(3):592–594

44. Jaeger HJ, Schmitz-Stolbrink A, Mathias KD. Cervical diastematomyelia and syringohydromyelia in a myelomeningocele patient. Eur Radiol 1997;7(4):477–479

45. Andro C, Pecquery R, De Vries P, Forlodou P, Fenoll B. Split cervical spinal cord malformation and vertebral dysgenesis. Orthop Traumatol Surg Res 2009;95(7):547–550

46. Maloney PR, Murphy ME, Sullan MJ, et al. Clinical and surgical management of a congenital Type II split cord malformation presenting with progressive cranial neuropathies: case report. J Neurosurg Pediatr 2017;19(3):349–353

47. Myles LM, Steers AJ, Minns R. Cervical cord tethering due to split cord malformation at the cervico-dorsal junction presenting with self-mutilation of the fingers. Dev Med Child Neurol 2002;44(12):844–848

48. Sonigo-Cohen P, Schmit P, Zerah M, et al. Prenatal diagnosis of diastematomyelia. Childs Nerv Syst 2003;19(7-8):555–560

49. Biri AA, Turp AB, Kurdoğlu M, Himmetoğlu O, Tokgöz Ercan N, Balci S. Prenatal diagnosis of diastematomyelia in a 15-week-old fetus. Fetal Diagn Ther 2005;20(4):258–261

50. Li SL, Luo G, Norwitz ER, et al. Prenatal diagnosis of diastematomyelia: a case report and review of the literature. J Clin Ultrasound 2012;40(5):301–305

51. Turgal M, Ozyuncu O, Talim B, Yazicioglu A, Onderoglu L. Prenatal diagnosis and clinicopathologic examination of a case with diastematomyelia. Congenit Anom (Kyoto) 2013;53(4):163–165

52. Lituania M, Tonni G, Araujo Júnior E. First trimester diagnosis of cervico-thoracic diastematomyelia and diplomyelia using three-dimensional ultrasound. Childs Nerv Syst 2015;31(12):2245–2248

53. Pérez LM, Barnes N, MacDiarmid SA, Oakes WJ, Webster GD. Urological dysfunction in patients with diastematomyelia. J Urol 1993;149(6):1503–1505

54. Proctor MR, Scott RM. Long-term outcome for patients with split cord malformation. Neurosurg Focus 2001;10(1):e5

55. Frerebeau P, Dimeglio A, Gras M, Harbi H. Diastematomyelia: report of 21 cases surgically treated by a neurosurgical and orthopedic team. Childs Brain 1983;10(5):328–339

56. McMaster MJ. Occult intraspinal anomalies and congenital scoliosis. J Bone Joint Surg Am 1984;66(4):588–601

57. Zuccaro G. Split spinal cord malformation. Childs Nerv Syst 2003;19(2):104–105

58. Matson DD, Woods RP, Campbell JB, Ingraham FD. Diastematomyelia (congenital clefts of the spinal cord); diagnosis and surgical treatment. Pediatrics 1950;6(1):98–112

59. Gilmor RL, Batnitzky S. Diastematomyelia—rare and unusual features. Neuroradiology 1978;16:87–88

60. Pang D, Parrish RG. Regrowth of diastematomyelic bone spur after extradural resection. Case report. J Neurosurg 1983;59(5):887–890

61. Gupta DK, Ahmed S, Garg K, Mahapatra AK. Regrowth of septal spur in split cord malformation. Pediatr Neurosurg 2010;46(3):242–244

62. Prasad GL, Borkar SA, Satyarthee GD, Mahapatra AK. Split cord malformation with dorsally located bony spur: report of four cases and review of literature. J Pediatr Neurosci 2012;7(3):167–170

63. Pang D. Split cord malformation: Part II: Clinical syndrome. Neurosurgery 1992;31(3):481–500

Composite Split Cord Malformations or Multisite Split Cord Malformations

Kanwaljeet Garg, Hitesh Inder Singh Rai, and Pankaj K. Singh

Table of Contents

■ Introduction 81

■ Complex Dysraphic Spine 81

■ Composite Split Cord Malformations 81

■ Incidence 82

■ Embryogenesis 82

■ Clinical Significance 83

■ Distribution of Spurs in Reported Cases 83

■ Cases Reported 83

■ Clinical Findings 84

■ Single Stage Surgery and Challenges 84

■ Conclusion 85

Composite Split Cord Malformations or Multisite Split Cord Malformations

Kanwaljeet Garg, Hitesh Inder Singh Rai, and Pankaj K. Singh

Introduction

Split cord malformations (SCMs) are an uncommon form of spinal dysraphism. The spinal cord is divided to form two neural tubes in SCM.[1-3] The length and number of places where the spinal cord is split varies significantly among cases. These malformations result due to abnormalities during early embryonic period (2–6 weeks of gestational age).[4] Early embryonic period is divided into three periods—gastrulation period (2nd to 3rd week), primary neurulation period (3rd week), and the secondary neurulation period (3rd to 4th week). Diastematomyelia and neurenteric cyst result from disorders of gastrulation, while meningocele and myelomeningocele arise from abnormalities of primary neurulation.[4] Conus and filum region abnormalities arise as a result of secondary neurulation disorders.[4] The fact that we get to see so many rare combinations of dysraphic abnormalities and so many variations in a single entity emphasizes the complexity of the underlying embryological processes,[1,4-14] which cannot be explained by simplified theory put by Pang et al in 1992.[15]

Complex Dysraphic Spine

Patnaik and Mahapatra defined complex dysraphic forms as "the conditions where there is more than one type of spinal dysraphism in the same patient involving various phases of embryogenesis."[4] These include more than one type of lesions present in one patient at one or different locations, or multiple similar type of lesions present at different locations in the same patient. They usually arise when multiple developmental periods are affected. They may or may not be associated with Chiari malformations, syrinx or hydrocephalus. However, any malformation arising during the gastrulation period is termed as a complex dysraphic state from the radiological perspective[4] (**Fig. 8.1**).

Composite Split Cord Malformations

Composite SCM is a type of complex spinal dysraphic abnormality. In composite SCM, there is single or different type of SCM in the same patient separated by intervening normal cord. SCM type I are characterized by a bony septum dividing the spinal canal into two halves, with two hemicords covered by a separate dural sheath, while the septum is fibrous and a single dural sheath cover for the hemicords in type II SCM.[15,16] Rest of the discussion in this chapter pertains to composite split cord malformations.

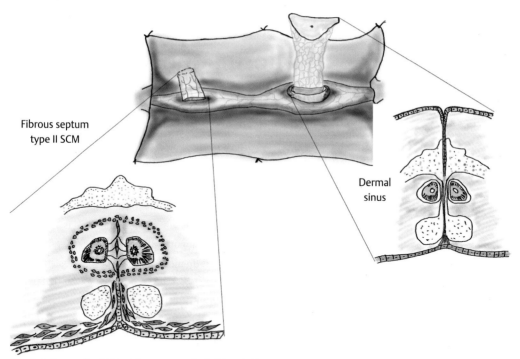

Fig. 8.1 A complex SCM with a type II split (left) with fibrous septum and a dermal sinus associated with a type I split (right).

Incidence

The true incidence of composite SCM is not known, as most of the reports come in the form of case reports only.[9,10,17–22] Harwood-Nash and McHugh reported that the incidence of composite SCM is less than 1%.[23] Erşahin reported 6 cases of composite SCM in his personal series of 131 patients.[18] Another surgeon reported only 2 cases of composite-type SCM out of a total of 39 cases in his series.[16] None of the other large series mention the incidence of composite SCM.[24,25] It emphasizes that composite SCM are grossly underreported.

Embryogenesis

Origin of composite-type SCM can be explained by multiple neurenteric canal theory, that is, multiple separate foci of ectoendodermal adhesions and endomesenchymal tracts, leading to development of SCM with intervening normal cord in the same patient.[9,16] The accessory neurenteric canal, which may be single or multiple, is the cause of SCM as per Pang's unified theory of embryogenesis. The presence of multiple accessory neurenteric canals results in two or more septa that form the endomesenchymal tracts and divide the neural tube resulting into two hemicords[9] (**Fig. 8.2**).

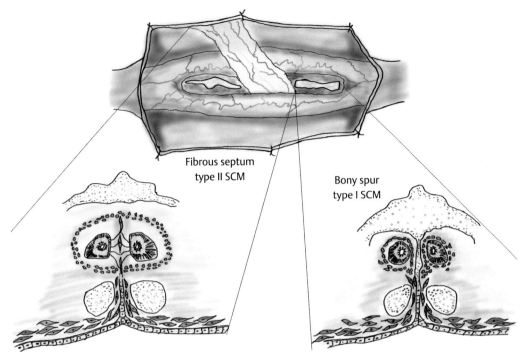

Fig. 8.2 A composite SCM with two type I splits interspersed by a type II split.

Clinical Significance

Composite SCM is rare but this fact should not preclude a neurosurgeon from performing whole spine MRI to find split at multiple locations, as missing SCM might be devastating for the patient.

Distribution of Spurs in Reported Cases

Most of these cases had two spurs at different levels, and one case having two different types of spurs at three different levels.[9,10] In most of these cases, the spurs were not more than three vertebral levels apart. Only one case had widely separated spurs present at T2 and L3 levels.[6,9,10,26] The spur is most commonly found in the lower thoracic or the upper lumbar region, and only four case reports of septum above T3 are available in the published literature (**Fig. 8.3**).

Cases Reported

Ailawadhi and Mahapatra reported a unique case of composite SCM, where the patient had three posterior bony spurs and one fibrous spur at different levels.[20] Khandelwal et al reported a case where the patient had a dorsal nonterminal myelocystocele, two level SCM type I and single level SCM type II,

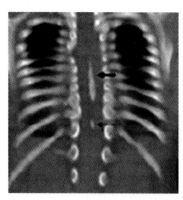

Fig. 8.3 CT scan coronal reconstruction showing two different bony spurs (the rostral one extending from D5 to D9 and the caudal one at D11).

hydrocephalus and coccygeal dermal sinus. The patient was operated for all the pathologies in one sitting (8-hour long surgery). The patient had good outcome with motor power in lower limbs same as in the preoperative period.

Vaishya and Jain reported three cases of composite-type SCM.[21] Akay et al reported a rare composite-type SCM of two different types at three different levels in the same patient.[9]

Singh et al reported a case of a long-segment type I SCM with two-level SCM and a single dural sac at the lower split.[22]

Akhtar et al reposted a case of two level type I SCM at thoracic level with dermal sinus tract, extradural dermoid cyst and an epidural abscess (**Table 8.1**).[17]

Clinical Findings

Presence of cutaneous stigma like hairy patch, capillary hemangioma should raise suspicion for SCM. Hypertrichosis is the most common cutaneous finding in patients with SCM and is seen in 20 to 55% of patients. The location of hypertrichosis correlates well with the location of SCM.[27] This type of SCM is rare, but this fact should not preclude a neurosurgeon from performing whole spine MRI to find split at multiple locations as missing SCM might be devastating for the patient (**Box 8.1**).

Single Stage Surgery and Challenges

Possible complications of single stage surgery at multiple locations include massive blood loss hypothermia, especially in young children. Both of these can result in significant postoperative morbidity. However, there are reports of dealing with these multiple abnormalities in single stage with good outcome.[10]

There are many challenges in the surgery of composite split cord malformation. The duration of surgery increases with the increasing number of levels being operated upon. The blood loss increases as well with the long/multiple incisions. The chances of neurological deterioration are also increased with the greater number of levels. No difference in the outcome of single spur or multiple spurs has been reported in literature. Singh et al reported good outcome at 6 months' follow up.[22]

Table 8.1 Summary of cases of composite split cord malformation published in literature

Year	Authors	Age/sex	Presentation
2001	Vaishya and Jain et al[21]	30 m/M	• Type II SCM at T7 and T10–T11 • Severe kyphoscoliosis in dorsal region and hyperpigmented patch on back
2001	Vaishya and Jain et al[21]	16 m/F	• Type I SCM at L2-L3 and Type II at L5 • Thoracic scoliosis
2001	Vaishya and Jain et al[21]	30 m/M	• Types I and II at L1–L3 • Thoracolumbar kyphoscoliosis and hypertrichosis
2005	Akay et al[9]	6 m/F	• Type I SCM at T4 and T5 • Type II SCM at T12 • Thoracic scoliosis with hypertrichosis
2011	Ailawadhi and Mahapatra[20]		• Type I SCM at T6, T12, and L3 • Thoracic scoliosis
2011	Khandelwal et al[10]		• Thoracic nonterminal myelocystocele at D7–D8 • Type II SCM at T10 • Type I SCM at L2–L3 • Dermal sinus in coccygeal region • Hydrocephalus
2012	Singh et al[19]		• Type II SCM at T2 • Type I SCM at L2 • Clubfeet • Hyperpigmented skin in upper thoracic and lower lumbar region with hypertrichosis and tenderness
2015	Akhtar et al[17]		• Type I SCM from T4 to T6 • Type I SCM from T9 to T11 • Dermoid cyst, Dermal sinus tract • Hypertrichosis

---

Box 8.1 Associated anomalies with complex SCM

- Skin stigmata: Hypertrichosis, capillary hemangioma, hyperpigmentation
- Dermoid cyst
- Dermal sinus tract
- Kyphoscoliosis
- Myelocystocele
- Hydrocephalus, syrinx
- Club feet

Conclusion

Composite SCM refers to a congenital condition in which there is a single or different type of SCMs in the same patient, separated by intervening normal cord. It is a rare anomaly. Surgery is challenging as the operative time and blood loss increases.

References

1. Garg K, Singh PK, Kale SS, Sharma BS. Long segment bony spur in split cord malformation type 1. Indian J Pediatr 2017;84(3):246–248

2. Bentley JF, Smith JR. Developmental posterior enteric remnants and spinal malformations: the split notochord syndrome. Arch Dis Child 1960;35:76–86

3. Laale HW. Ethanol induced notochord and spinal cord duplications in the embryo of the zebrafish, Brachydanio rerio. J Exp Zool 1971;177(1):51–64

4. Patnaik A, Mahapatra AK. Complex forms of spinal dysraphism. Childs Nerv Syst 2013;29(9): 1527–1532

5. Garg K, Mahapatra AK, Tandon V. A rare case of type 1 C split cord malformation with single dural sheath. Asian J Neurosurg 2015;10(3):226–228

6. Garg K, Tandon V, Mahapatra AK. A unique case of split cord malformation type 1 with three different types of bony spurs. Asian J Neurosurg 2017;12(2):305–308

7. Garg K, Kumar R. Complex spinal dysraphism with multiple anomalies. Pediatr Neurosurg 2013;49(2):126–128

8. Garg K, Kumar R. Complex split cord malformation type 1 with multiple lipomas involving the split cord. Pediatr Neurosurg 2013;49(2):121–123

9. Akay KM, Izci Y, Baysefer A, Timurkaynak E. Composite type of split cord malformation: two different types at three different levels: case report. J Neurosurg 2005; 102(4, Suppl):436–438

10. Khandelwal A, Tandon V, Mahapatra AK. An unusual case of 4 level spinal dysraphism: Multiple composite type 1 and type 2 split cord malformation, dorsal myelocystocele and hydrocephalous. J Pediatr Neurosci 2011;6(1):58–61

11. Garg K, Tandon V, Gupta DK, Sharma BS. Multiple neural tube defect with split cord malformation: a rare entity. Indian J Pediatr 2014;81(9):982–983

12. van Aalst J, Beuls EA, Vles JS, Cornips EM, van Straaten HW. The intermediate type split cord malformation: hypothesis and case report. Childs Nerv Syst 2005;21(12):1020–1024

13. Solanki GA, Evans J, Copp A, Thompson DNP. Multiple coexistent dysraphic pathologies. Childs Nerv Syst 2003;19(5–6):376–379

14. Dhandapani S, Srinivasan A. Contiguous triple spinal dysraphism associated with Chiari malformation Type II and hydrocephalus: an embryological conundrum between the unified theory of Pang and the unified theory of McLone. J Neurosurg Pediatr 2016;17(1):103–106

15. Pang D, Dias MS, Ahab-Barmada M. Split cord malformation: part I—a unified theory of embryogenesis for double spinal cord malformations. Neurosurgery 1992;31(3):451–480

16. Pang D. Split cord malformation: part II—clinical syndrome. Neurosurgery 1992;31(3):481–500

17. Akhtar S, Azeem A, Shamim MS, Tahir MZ. Composite split cord malformation associated with a dermal sinus tract, dermoid cyst, and epidural abscess: a case report and review of literature. Surg Neurol Int 2016;7:43

18. Erşahin Y. Split cord malformation types I and II: a personal series of 131 patients. Childs Nerv Syst 2013;29(9):1515–1526

19. Singh DK, Singh N, Singh R. Widely separated composite split cord malformation. BMJ Case Rep 2012;2012:bcr2012007028

20. Ailawadhi P, Mahapatra AK. An unusual case of spinal dysraphism with four splits including three posterior spurs. Pediatr Neurosurg 2011;47(5):372–375

21. Vaishya S, Kumarjain P. Split cord malformation: three unusual cases of composite split cord malformation. Childs Nerv Syst 2001;17(9):528–530

22. Singh PK, Khandelwal A, Singh A, Ailawadhi P, Gupta D, Mahapatra AK. Long-segment type 1 split cord malformation with two-level split cord malformation and a single dural sac at the lower split. Pediatr Neurosurg 2011;47(3):227–229

23. Harwood-Nash DC, McHugh K. Diastematomyelia in 172 children: the impact of modern neuroradiology. Pediatr Neurosurg 1990–1991;16(4-5):247–251

24. Mahapatra AK, Gupta DK. Split cord malformations: a clinical study of 254 patients and a proposal for a new clinical-imaging classification. J Neurosurg 2005;103(6, Suppl)531–536

25. Sinha S, Agarwal D, Mahapatra AK. Split cord malformations: an experience of 203 cases. Childs Nerv Syst 2006;22(1):3–7

26. McClelland RR, Marsh DG. Double diastematomyelia. Radiology 1977;123(2):378

27. Higashida T, Sasano M, Sato H, Sekido K, Ito S. Myelomeningocele associated with split cord malformation type I: three case reports. Neurol Med Chir (Tokyo) 2010;50(5):426–430

Adult Split Cord Malformations

Mohit Agrawal, Manoj Phalak, and Ashok K. Mahapatra

Table of Contents

■ Introduction 91

■ Pathophysiology 91

■ Demography 91

■ Clinical Features 95

■ Imaging 96

■ Treatment and Outcome 96

■ Conclusion 97

Adult Split Cord Malformations

Mohit Agrawal, Manoj Phalak, and Ashok K. Mahapatra

Introduction

Split cord malformation (SCM) is predominantly a diagnosis of childhood which presents in a varied manner. In recent years, this entity has been diagnosed in adults as well. This has been partly due to improved imaging and recognition of this condition. In a literature review published in 1990, Russel et al identified 45 adult cases with diastematomyelia.[1] Since then, the number of case reports with adult SCM have grown considerably, with most case series of adult tethered cord syndrome (TCS) reporting patients with this form of spinal dysraphism. The benefit of early surgical detethering in children has been well-established in literature. There is a lack of clarity as far as the clinical and management aspects of adult SCM is concerned, which is still controversial with regard to asymptomatic patients, who are incidentally diagnosed with this condition.

Pathophysiology

The reason why children with TCS develop neurological deterioration is because of the stretching and consequent injury to the nerve fibers as the child grows. Adults have already completed their growth curve and somehow not developed any symptoms despite the presence of tethering element caudally. However, the risk of neurological deficits occurring due to mechanical stretching of the spine during trauma or any specific postures is still present. It has also been seen that patients might ignore or downplay long-standing minor neurological deficits and not seek any medical help for the same.[2] Patients with progressive scoliosis or those with degenerative spine[3] may become symptomatic as the configuration of the spine changes. Another set of patients in which adult SCM has been reported are those in whom scoliosis correction surgery was performed when they belonged to the adolescent age group, that is, before the widespread use of MRI as a screening tool to look for TCS prior to surgery.[4] These patients present in adulthood with progressive neurological deterioration.

Demography

Adult SCM has predominantly been reported in females (**Table 9.1**). Russel et al[1] in a review on all the case reports on adult SCM found 45 patients with a F:M ratio of 3.4:1. The cause of this gender predilection is unknown. This condition presents in a wide age group, ranging from 18 to 88 years,[5] with no definite peak in any decade.

Table 9.1 Management and outcomes reported in world literature on adult SCM

Author	No. of patients	Age and gender	Cord ending/type of split and level	Surgery	Complication	Follow-up/postop status
Shukla et al[6]	7	Not mentioned separately	2– type I, 5– type II (level not mentioned)	Detethering with removal of spur	NA	Improved or stable
Viswanathan et al[7]	2	67/F	L4/L2–3 type II spur, T12 syrinx	Laminectomy + removal of spur with detethering	None	5.5 years/improved
		53/F	L3/type I spur at L1–2	Laminectomy + removal of spur with detethering	None	1 year/improved
Davanzo et al[8]	1	43/M	L5/Duplicated filum terminale	Laminectomy and detethering	Pseudomeningocele– re-exploration and repair	6 weeks/improved
Kim et al[9]	1	34/F	L5/C7–D11 type II spur	Laminectomy + removal of spur with detethering	None	7 years/improvement (pain and motor)
Borkar et al[10]	7	Not mentioned separately	M/c thoracic f/b lumbar (level not mentioned)	Laminectomy + removal of spur with detethering	7% patients had long-term deficits	Improvement/stable
Klekamp[11]	24	46 ± 13 years (range 23–74 years)	22– lumbar, 2– cervical	Detethering and spur removal	NA	Improvement/stable
Rahimizadeh et al[12]	1	72/F	C5–D3 type I spur	None	NA	18 months/stable
Conti et al[13]	2	87/M	Intramedullary dermoid cyst with type II spur at L1	Laminectomy and excision of tumor	None	1 month/improvement (pain and sensorimotor)
		38/F	L1–2 intramedullary teratoma with type II spur	Laminectomy and excision of tumor	None	2 months/improvement (pain)
Méndez et al[5]	1	88/F	L2–5 type I spur with L4 vertebral body collapse	L4 vertebroplasty	NA	Improvement (pain)

Table 9.1 *Continued*

Table 9.1 (*Continued*) Management and outcomes reported in world literature on adult SCM

Author	No. of patients	Age and gender	Cord ending/type of split and level	Surgery	Complication	Follow-up/postop status
Armstrong et al[14]	1	37/F	D1 type II spur	NA	NA	NA
Porensky et al[15]	1	54/F	L4, D4–D9, D11–L3 type II spur, type I spur at D8, D7–8 extramedullary epidermoid cyst	Laminectomy + removal of spur with tumor excision	Pulmonary embolism	8 months/improvement (pain, sensorimotor, sphincter deficits with stable scoliosis)
Guilloton et al[16]	2	40/F	Type II spur at L2	None	NA	NA
		54/F	Type II spur D12–L1	None	NA	NA
Goina et al[17]	1	68/F	L4, type II spur at L2 with cranial syrinx	NA	NA	NA
Lewandrowski et al[4]	1	44/F	L1–2 type I spur	Laminectomy with removal of fusion mass and spur	Pseudomeningocele	1 year/improvement
Pallatroni et al[18]	1	78/F	L5, L3–4 type II spur	None	None	NA
Soni et al[19]	1	30/F	D7–8 type I SCM with extramedullary neuroenteric cyst	Laminectomy + excision of bony spur and cyst	None	3 month/improvement
Quinones-Hinojosa et al[3]	1	73/F	L3/type II spur D12–L3	Laminectomy + removal of spur with detethering	None	6 weeks/improvement (pain and motor)
Sheehan et al[20]	1	38/F	D1–D3 type II spur, D2–4 intramedullary epidermoid, cranial syrinx	Laminectomy + removal of spur with tumor excision	None	Improvement (pain, sensorimotor, sphincter deficits)
Hüttmann et al[21]	12	Not mentioned separately	Not mentioned separately	NA	NA	8 years (mean)/improvement/stable

Table 9.1 *Continued*

Table 9.1 *(Continued)* Management and outcomes reported in world literature on adult SCM

Author	No. of patients	Age and gender	Cord ending/type of split and level	Surgery	Complication	Follow-up/postop status
Wenger et al[22]	1	38/F	L3–4 level type II spur	None	NA	Improved on conservative management
Kaminker et al[23]	1	38/M	L4/ type I spur L2–3	Laminectomy + extradural removal of spur	None	2 years/improvement (pain)
Iskandar et al[2]	13	Mean–34 years	Not mentioned separately	NA	NA	Improvement/stable
Prasad et al[24]	2	28/M	L4–5 type I spur	Laminectomy + removal of spur with detethering	None	Improvement (pain and sensorimotor)
		22/F	D11–12 type I spur	Laminectomy and spur excision	None	Improvement (pain and urinary symptoms)
Pang[25]	8	Not mentioned separately	6–type I, 2–type II spur	NA	NA	NA
Russell et al[1]–review article of all previous reported cases	45	19–76 (mean–37.8 years), 3.4:1 F:M	M/C lumbar	24 patients underwent surgery	NA	23 showed improvement

Abbreviation: SCM, split cord malformation.

Clinical Features

Backache is the most common presenting complaint in adult SCM (**Fig. 9.1**). It may present with or without features of radiculopathy in the distribution of the involved nerve roots.[6,8,13,15,16,18–20,24] For most adults, this may be the only complaint, with the pathology being found upon investigation into the cause of the pain. Adults present with some mild form of sensorimotor deficits or bladder symptoms. Unlike the pediatric population where these symptoms are investigated earlier, adults tend to ignore the symptoms attributing it to some other cause. The lack of knowledge about this condition, amongst patients and doctors, is the reason for some of the cases of late diagnosis of this condition in the 7th and

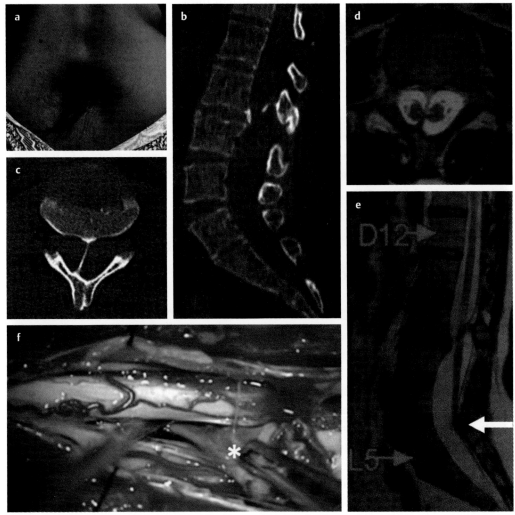

Fig. 9.1 A 23-year-old female presented with a history of progressive low backache for the past 4 years. She had no urinary complaints and had no neurological deficits. **(a)** Local examination showed hypertrichosis over the lower back. **(b, c)** CT scan of the lumbosacral spine showed a L2-L3 bony spur. **(d, e)** MRI confirmed the diagnosis of Type I SCM with low lying cord at L5 (arrow). She underwent laminectomy, spur removal and detethering of the low-lying cord. **(f)** Intraoperative image showing the split cords with the bony spur being removed (asterisk). She had an uneventful postoperative period and is doing well at follow up.

8th decades, despite the patient having obvious cutaneous markers or musculoskeletal deformity. Hypertrichosis[6-8,13,24,25] is the most common associated cutaneous marker reported in adult SCM, followed by dermal sinus.[6,17] Orthopedic abnormalities like scoliosis or club foot are less commonly found in adult SCM, with most patients with these conditions being diagnosed and managed appropriately in childhood itself. Development of new deficits, or the progression of minor established ones, finally lead these patients to seek medical attention in late adulthood.[2]

There are many case reports of incidental diagnosis of the condition following trauma,[1] symptoms aggravated during pregnancy,[19] or following spinal anesthesia.[22] It might sometimes even be associated with tumors like teratoma/epidermoid/dermoid cyst/neuroenteric cyst,[15,19,20] with mixed clinical features of an intradural/intramedullary compression along with tethering.

The level of the split is most commonly found in the lumbar or lower dorsal regions, with rare case reports in the upper dorsal[9,14,15,19,20] or cervical region.[11,12]

Imaging

High-resolution MRI is the imaging modality of choice, which delineates the split, tethering element, and the position of the hemicords clearly. A whole spine MRI should be obtained to rule out the presence of associated anomalies like syrinx, Chiari malformation, tumors, or a low-lying cord. A CT scan of the region with the split is important to visualize the complete extent, the attachment, and the direction of the bony spur (**Fig. 9.1**).

Other investigative modalities like uroflowmetry and ultrasound abdomen are complementary to document the preoperative deficits and objective evaluation of any change in symptoms after surgery.

Treatment and Outcome

The various management strategies and their outcomes reported in world literature are summarized in **Table 9.1**.

Surgical intervention is recommended if there is a new onset neurological deficit or progression of pre-existing neurological deficits. The most common symptom to be relieved is pain, with almost all reports showing improvement postoperatively. The next most common neurological deficit to be either stabilized or show improvement is sensorimotor symptoms, with only few case reports of neurogenic bladder improvement. Surgical procedure of choice is similar to pediatric cases with laminectomy, complete spur removal, and detethering of low-lying cord. Few case reports of only spur removal without detethering of cord are present in literature, although without long-term follow-up of these patients, such partial procedures are not recommended. Intraoperative neuromonitoring is an invaluable tool in order to minimize postoperative neurological deficits and the prompt recognition of any iatrogenic injury during the procedure.[26,27]

Management of patients in whom this condition is detected incidentally or those with a long-standing fixed neurological deficit is debatable. Due to the limited case reports of such patients, a clear notion of the natural history of the disease is not known.

Klekamp[11] in his study on long-term follow-up of 84 adult tethered cord patients, out of which 24 were SCM, recommended that surgery should be performed in symptomatic patients only. He proposed a conservative approach in patients without any neurological deficits. All the patients in this study who underwent revision surgery for complex dysraphic lesions eventually deteriorated, and he advised caution in their management.

Hüttmann et al[21] analyzed 54 patients with adult tethered cord (12 SCM) and identified two risk factors associated with a poor outcome. One was the presence of preoperative neurological deficits for more than 5 years. The other was an evidence of incomplete detethering. Eight out of 10 such patients in their study developed recurrent symptoms 5 years after surgery compared to only seven out of 44 patients (16%) in whom complete detethering was performed.

Shukla et al[6] compared outcomes of pediatric and adult TCS at their center. They found that adult spinal dysraphisms constituted 15.4% of their patients, with SCM being the second most common diagnosis in adults after lipomeningocele. They also found that the most common symptom to improve following detethering in adult TCS was pain followed by motor weakness.

Conclusion

Adult SCM remains a rare condition. Knowledge about this condition and clinical suspicion in the mind of treating physicians is necessary to diagnose this condition early. Any adult patient presenting with neurocutaneous stigmata of dysraphism should be properly evaluated. Imaging of adults with low backache should also be studied thoroughly to look for low-lying cord or SCM. Surgical treatment of symptomatic patients with neurological deterioration is mandatory. Many factors such as age and associated comorbidities need to be considered before prescribing surgery for asymptomatic patients or those with mild backache. Surgical intervention is recommended in order to preserve the remaining neurological function or to attempt a partial recovery of the same.

References

1. Russell NA, Benoit BG, Joaquin AJ. Diastematomyelia in adults: a review. Pediatr Neurosurg 1990–1991;16(4-5):252–257
2. Iskandar BJ, Fulmer BB, Hadley MN, Oakes WJ. Congenital tethered spinal cord syndrome in adults. J Neurosurg 1998;88(6):958–961
3. Quinones-Hinojosa A, Gadkary CA, Mummaneni PV, Rosenberg WS. Split spinal cord malformation in an elderly patient: case report. Surg Neurol 2004;61(2):201–203
4. Lewandrowski KU, Rachlin JR, Glazer PA. Diastematomyelia presenting as progressive weakness in an adult after spinal fusion for adolescent idiopathic scoliosis. Spine J 2004;4(1):116–119
5. Méndez JC, Prieto MA, Lanciego C. Percutaneous vertebroplasty in a patient with type I split cord malformation (diastematomyelia). Cardiovasc Intervent Radiol 2009;32(3):608–610
6. Shukla M, Sardhara J, Sahu RN, et al. Adult versus pediatric tethered cord syndrome: clinicoradiological differences and its management. Asian J Neurosurg 2018;13(2):264–270
7. Viswanathan VK, Minnema AJ, Farhadi HF. Surgical management of adult type 1 split cord malformation. Report of two cases with literature review. J Clin Neurosci 2018;52:119–121
8. Davanzo JR, Christopher Zacko J, Specht CS, Rizk EB. Duplicate filum terminale noted in an adult: a rare finding. J Neurosurg Spine 2016;25(3):415–417

9. Kim YD, Sung JH, Hong JT, Lee SW. Split cord malformation combined with tethered cord syndrome in an adult. J Korean Neurosurg Soc 2013;54(4):363–365

10. Borkar SA, Mahapatra AK. Split cord malformations: a two years experience at AIIMS. Asian J Neurosurg 2012;7(2):56–60

11. Klekamp J. Tethered cord syndrome in adults. J Neurosurg Spine 2011;15(3):258–270

12. Rahimizadeh A, Kaghazchi M. Cervicothoracic diastematomyelia in an elderly with normal neurology: report of a case and review of the literature. World Spinal Column Journal 2011;2(2):68–72

13. Conti P, Tenenbaum R, Capozza M, Mouchaty H, Conti R. Diastematomyelia and tumor in adults: report of two cases and literature review. Spine 2010;35(24):E1438–E1443

14. Armstrong DJ, Chadwick L, Finch MB. Diastematomyelia presenting with neck stiffness. Clin Rheumatol 2007;26(3):451

15. Porensky P, Muro K, Ganju A. Adult presentation of spinal dysraphism and tandem diastematomyelia. Spine J 2007;7(5):622–626

16. Guilloton L, Allary M, Jacquin O, et al. Split-cord malformation (diastematolmyelia) presenting in two adults: case report and a review of the literature. Rev Neurol (Paris) 2004;160(12):1180–1186

17. Goina LS, Verstichel P, Roualdès B, El Amrani M, Meyrignac C. Type II split cord malformation of late clinical onset. Rev Neurol (Paris) 2004;160(1):86–88

18. Pallatroni HF, Ball PA, Duhaime AC. Split cord malformation as a cause of tethered cord syndrome in a 78-year-old female. Pediatr Neurosurg 2004;40(2):80–83

19. Soni TV, Pandya C, Vaidya JP. Split cord malformation with neurenteric cyst and pregnancy. Surg Neurol 2004;61(6):556–558

20. Sheehan JP, Sheehan JM, Lopes MB, Jane JA Sr. Thoracic diastematomyelia with concurrent intradural epidermoid spinal cord tumor and cervical syrinx in an adult: case report. J Neurosurg 2002; 97(2, Suppl):231–234

21. Hüttmann S, Krauss J, Collmann H, Sörensen N, Roosen K. Surgical management of tethered spinal cord in adults: report of 54 cases. J Neurosurg 2001; 95(2, Suppl):173–178

22. Wenger M, Hauswirth CB, Brodhage RP. Undiagnosed adult diastematomyelia associated with neurological symptoms following spinal anaesthesia. Anaesthesia 2001;56(8):764–767

23. Kaminker R, Fabry J, Midha R, Finkelstein JA. Split cord malformation with diastematomyelia presenting as neurogenic claudication in an adult: a case report. Spine 2000;25(17):2269–2271

24. Prasad VS, Sengar RL, Sahu BP, Immaneni D. Diastematomyelia in adults. Modern imaging and operative treatment. Clin Imaging 1995;19(4):270–274

25. Pang D. Split cord malformation: Part II: Clinical syndrome. Neurosurgery 1992;31(3):481–500

26. Quiñones-Hinojosa A, Gadkary CA, Gulati M, et al. Neurophysiological monitoring for safe surgical tethered cord syndrome release in adults. Surg Neurol 2004;62(2):127–133

27. Paradiso G, Lee GY, Sarjeant R, Hoang L, Massicotte EM, Fehlings MG. Multimodality intraoperative neurophysiologic monitoring findings during surgery for adult tethered cord syndrome: analysis of a series of 44 patients with long-term follow-up. Spine 2006;31(18):2095–2102

Complex Split Cord Malformations

Shweta Kedia, Ramesh Doddamani, and Ashok K. Mahapatra

Table of Contents

- **Introduction** 101

- **Embryogenesis** 102

- **Clinical Presentation** 105

- **Investigations** 105

- **Treatment** 106

- **Conclusion** 107

Complex Split Cord Malformations

Shweta Kedia, Ramesh Doddamani, and Ashok K. Mahapatra

Introduction

Congenital malformations in spine may present at birth or may be discovered late in life. In actual clinical practice, it is not rare to find an amalgam of disorders which defies any embryological explanation. Several attempts have been made to simplify the classification system in order to establish a uniformity in reporting. One such attempt was made by Tortori et al who tried to devise a new cliniconeuroradiological classification for children with spinal dysraphism.[1] Their classification system described the closed dysraphism and one of the subtypes was complex dysraphic states. This state has been classically referred to as the disorders occurring in the gastrulation stage.[2] Thus, the clinical spectrum covered under complex dysraphic states is listed below:

- Dorsal enteric cysts.
- Neurenteric cysts.
- Split cord malformations (SCMs).
- Dermal sinus.
- Caudal regression syndrome.
- Segmental dysgenesis.

As per this classification, all SCMs belong to the complex dysraphic states. However, in clinical practice, we do come across patients with SCMs along with other dysraphism, open or closed. The best way to describe them would be to refer to them as "complex spina bifida." After a thorough literature search, we could find the term "complex spina bifida" first used by Raj Kumar et al in their paper on SCM with meningomyeloceles (MMC).[3,4] He preferred to classify them as a separate entity to understand their embryology and clinical implications better, and proposed a revised classification over that of Pang's as type I SCM with MMC and type II with MMC.[3]

Since then, the term "complex spinal dysraphism" have been used by several authors to illustrate the presence of multi- or same level, similar or different forms of spinal dysraphism, with or without hydrocephalus or syrinx, presenting in single individuals.[5-11] This definition is controversial and may extend to include anything that is beyond the definition of isolated spinal dysraphism.

Mahapatra et al made an attempt to classify these complex dysraphisms into five broad categories based on literature citations.[11]

The common complex SCM encountered in clinical practice are as follows:

- Complex spinal dysraphism.
- Multicomponent spinal dysraphisms, consisting variable combinations of myelomeningocele, SCMs, lipoma, neurenteric cyst, dermoid, etc.
- Multilevel spinal dysraphisms like SCMs.

- Complex lipoma.
- Spinal dysraphisms with Arnold–Chiari malformation with or without associated hydrocephalus and syringomyelia.
- Spinal dysraphisms associated with other organ system malformations.

Embryogenesis

Complex spinal dysraphism occurs due to the disorders occurring in early embryonic stage (2–6 weeks). This stage involves complex changes in the cellular arrangements in the embryo and consists of gastrulation (weeks 2–3), primary neurulation (week 3), and secondary neurulation (week 3–4) and then goes through a multistep process.[12,13] Any of the two stages with the gastrulation stage may be involved in complex dysraphisms. When the formation of the endomesenchymal tract happens before 3 weeks, it gives rise to type II SCM. SCM type I occurs when the endomesenchymal tract formation takes place after 4 weeks of gestation. The presence of commonly associated spinal abnormalities such as dermal sinus tracts, spinal lipomas, dermoids, neurenteric cysts, and even a meningocele or myelomeningocele occurs if the abnormal fistula forms between day 21 and 30.[14]

This form of presentation of SCM, while defies the universal theory of embryogenesis as advocated by Pang, also opens up the discussion on missing links between gastrulation and neurulation.[2,15] Despite the various embryological hypotheses that have been put forth to explain the etiology of different types of spinal dysraphism, the experimental evidence in support of the same is absent.[13,16–21] The discrete nature of the lesions in these cases do imply that there are multiple sites of embryogenetic error happening in different stages in a particular individual. So, in a patient with SCM with low-lying cord along with hydromyelia, spinal lipoma and MMC, varied embryological stages are being affected. Partial retrogressive differentiation along with failed terminal cord involution results in low-lying cord.[22] Abnormal dilatation of the central canal after neural tube closure causes hydromyelia.[23] When there is premature separation of ectoderm and neuroectoderm during neurulation, it results in spinal lipoma,[24] and MMC arises from failed neural-tube closure.

The overdistension theory has also been used to explain the extremely high occurrence of multiple neural tube defects in the same baby. Therefore, oversecretion of neural tube fluid leads to rupture of the closed neural tube, resulting in secondary neural tube defects.[25]

As per Gardner, rupture of this overexpanded neural tube beneath an intact cutaneous ectoderm results in the proteinaceous neural tube fluid infiltrating the mesoderm. This extraneous protein causes dislocation of cells and further injury occurs by yet unidentifiable substrates of mesodermal organs.

This would also explain the occurrence of composite SCM.

Each subtype of these complex forms of dysraphism have been well described in literature. A knowledge of all of these is important, so as not to get carried away by the more obvious anomaly and miss out on other hidden offending pathologies existing simultaneously. In order to discuss the complex dysraphism, we need to walk through the complete spectrum of its associations.

■ Multicomponent Complex Spinal Dysraphism

The first and foremost topic authors discuss is MMC, which is the most common concurrent finding with SCM. It is a classic example of a situation where both the closed and open forms of dysraphism coexist. Data on its incidence varies because of the lack of uniform reporting system, but almost 10 to 40% of the cases of SCM may present with MMC. They also frequently present along with Chiari malformation, hydrocephalus, and syrinx, which are not otherwise present in pure SCMs (**Fig. 10.1**).[3,26–28] Akiyama et al[29] and Yamanaka et al[30] have both reported cases on SCM with myeloschisis on separate occasions. Higashida et al documented absence of right kidney and hypoplastic sacrum in one of their MMC patients with SCM. There is also mention of hemimyelomeningocele in the literature, although rare.[31–33] It may also be associated with a neurenteric cyst (**Fig. 10.2**). Rowley and Johnson reported a case of lumbar SCMs where one cord failed to neurulate, resulting in hemimyelomeningocele and associated Chiari II malformation and other visceral and osseous anomalies.[32]

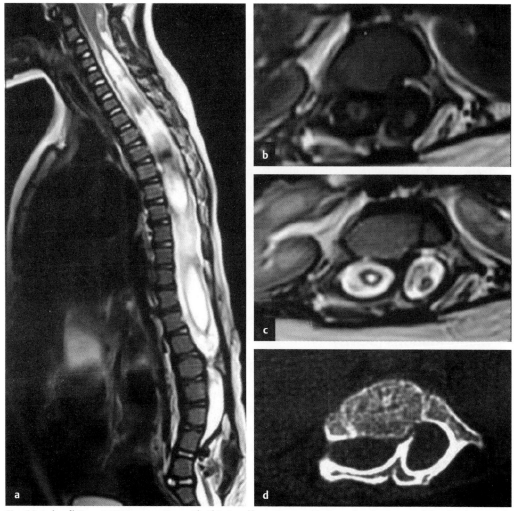

Fig. 10.1 (a–d) Type 1 SCM presenting with Chiari malformation and holocord syrinx is one of the classic example of complex dysraphism.

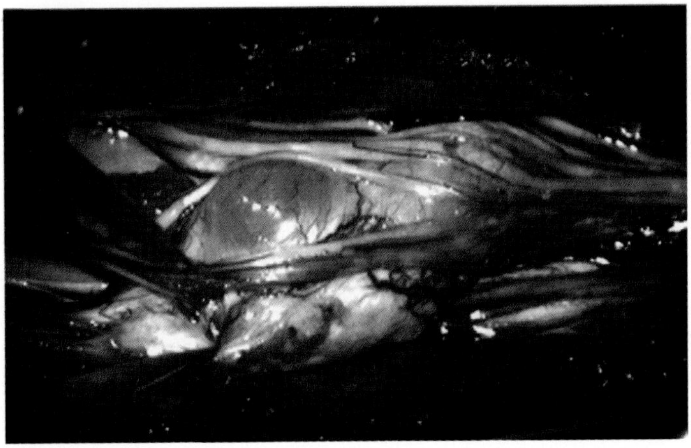

Fig. 10.2 Spinal dysraphism along with neurenteric cyst is another form of complex spinal dysraphism.

Myelocystocele has also been reported to coexist with SCM. Parmar et al first described terminal myelocystocele arising from one hemicord in a 4-month-old girl with SCM I.[34] This patient also had ectopic right kidney, Chiari I malformation, and partial sacral agenesis. Solanki et al reported a 10-month-old child with a type I SCM associated with hemivertebrae, lipomyelomeningoceles in each hemicord of the SCM, and a terminal myelocystocele.[19] This child was operated for myelocystocele elsewhere and the rest of the tethering elements were not looked for. The occurrence of all of this in one individual patient would require involvement of gastrulation, primary, as well as secondary neurulation. There are reports of nonterminal myelocystocele as well along with composite SCM.[35]

There have been several reports on multiple forms of dysraphism present at different levels in one individual. Emmez et al enumerated seven congenital malformations consisting of hydrocephalus, Chiari malformation, syringohydromyelia, SCM, dermal sinus tract, lumbosacral MMC, and tethered cord.[36] Similarly, Avcu et al reported a 5-year-old boy presenting with six different forms of dysraphism.[37] Maiti et al reported two cases of complex SCM with intraspinal teratoma, one located intramedullary and the other extradural within meningocele.[38] Naik et al and Ugarte et al reported a complex spinal dysraphism with mediastinal teratoma in two separate occasions.[39,40]

■ Multilevel Complex Spinal Dysraphism or Composite Split Cord Malformations (SCMs)

Moving away from the discussion of different spinal dysraphisms present in one patient to multilevel split in single individual with intervening normal cord, multiple neurenteric canal theory leading to two or more separate foci of ectoendodermal adhesions and endomesenchymal tracts can explain the embryology of composite SCM. The incidence, however, is exceptionally low, which may be because in the past, we were not looking for it. Harwood et al documented the frequency of composite SCM as 1%, while Pang et al had only two cases of composite SCM II in a cohort of 39 patients.[41,42] Ersahin reported four cases of composite SCM.[43] The literature thereafter does show an increasing frequency of this entity.[44–47] This gets further complicated when it is associated with other forms of spinal dysraphism. Jarmundowicz reported a case of composite SCM with spinal cord teratoma.[48]

■ Spinal Dysraphisms Associated with Other Organ System Malformations

The third broad category of complex spinal dysraphisms with significant clinical implications is the ones associated with anomalies of other organ systems. Situs inversus has been described by Dwarkanath et al and Tubbs et al on two separate occasions.[49,50] The anorectal malformation and omphalocele, exstrophy of the cloaca, imperforate anus, and spinal defects (OEIS) complex have also been described coexisting with dysraphisms in literature.[51,52] Shieh and Lam reported a 1-day-old male neonate presenting with multiple right-sided anomalies, including hypoplastic right face and decreased movement of the right upper extremity with absent right cervical hemivertebrae, right cervical lipomyelomeningocele, and cervical diplomyelia with right hemicord terminating in a blind pouch.[53]

Clinical Presentation

The overt clinical presentation of these patients is no different from the other open or closed dysraphisms. It obviously depends on what all dysraphic features exist along with each other and which other organ system is involved. High level of suspicion is needed when one first encounters a patient of congenital malformation, and a thorough search for all other associated anomalies need to be done. There will be variable motor, sensory, and bladder and bowel disturbances, depending on the amount of neural tissue involved and the level of lesion. One of the tell-tale signs of two pathologies in the same patient is the cutaneous stigma at two different sites. Patients may present with hairy patch, and capillary hemangioma over an area other than visible spina bifida aperta lesion. Quite contrary to our expectations, these cutaneous markers may be less evident in patients with MMC with SCM rather than pure SCM.[42,43]

The neurological deficits not getting explained by the lumbar MMC may be explained by the SCM at a higher level. Some clinical pointers could be unilateral paresis, hypertrichosis only on one side of the defect, or progressive scoliosis, which may provide clinical clues to the diagnosis.[54]

In his comparative study of MMC with SCM versus pure SCM or MMC, Kumar et al observed that the neurological dysfunctions were relatively more common in MMC patients with SCM than in only MMC patients, while neuro-orthopedic deformities were more frequent in only MMC group as compared to MMC with SCM group. More often than not, there may not be an obvious clinical cue to the underlying dual or more pathology. But often, the complex nature of the spinal malformation is clinically unsuspected.[55]

Needless to say, any patient of spinal dysraphism deserves a thorough local, neurological, and other systemic evaluation done.

Investigations

Meticulous imaging of patients with spinal dysraphisms is paramount. The fact these cases are seldom mentioned in the literature in the past is because of lack of screening MRI scans. In the authors' institute, they prefer to do a screening brain and MRI scan for all the patients with spinal dysraphisms. In cases of ruptured MMC, such patients would be taken to surgeries within first 48 hours and then would be investigated for other coexisting pathologies. This has helped them pick up several composite and complex forms of spinal dysraphism. There are reports to suggest the applicability of curved planar reformation (CPR) for evaluating hydromyelia in patients with scoliosis associated with spinal dysraphism. The authors used the constructive interference in steady state (CISS) sequence along with T1 and T2W MRI sequences and reformatted in two planes to assess the length and extent of spinal cord involvement.[56]

In his illustrative cases, Rauzzino et al describes 13 patients with neurenteric cyst along with other spinal dysraphism. They clearly found the usefulness of MRI in diagnosing and locating these cysts along with the other dysraphic features.[57]

As a part of surgical planning, 3D CT is routinely done along with MR imaging in patients with SCM. CT scan provides the detailed bony anatomy of the septum, their orientation, and extension, and MRI gives the details of the cord status.

Ultrasonography has been found useful as a noninvasive screening in infants up to 6 months of age before ossification of the vertebral bodies. The drawback of this imaging system, however, is that it is largely operator-dependent and less sensitive than MRI.[58,59]

Treatment

Identifying the coexisting pathology is the first step to treat these complex spinal dysraphisms. The surgeon should be aware of how many pathologies she or he is dealing with, what levels, and the steps to deal with them individually.

The surgical steps for the removal of bony spur remains the same, as described elsewhere. Few important practical points that the authors learned through experience are as follows:

1. Skin incision should be planned well in advance, taking into account the multilevels. It is not advisable to leave small strips of skin in between when the two levels are really close by. On the other hand, if they are further apart, two separate skin incision would minimize blood loss.

2. Opening the layers of skin and fascia to form a good plane. This gives one plenty of room to close the defects adequately later without fear of skin necrosis and cerebrospinal fluid (CSF) leak.

3. In case of bony split, authors tend to remove the spur first and then treat the MMC or low-lying conus.

4. Authors generally intend to start from top to bottom, so, for example, the lesions in the D6–8 will be tackled first, then D10, and then L2–3.

5. Most of the times adequate dural closure is achievable, if not, authors prefer to use the fascia in the paraspinal area. Watertight dura closure is a must.

6. Most of these surgeries have long incision and a subfascial drain may be placed at the time of closure. However, it is not a routine and depends on the surgeon's preference.

7. The first wound check is done only after 48 hours unless the wound is soaked. The suture removal can be done within a standard window of 8 to 10 days.

8. Finally, life-threatening diseases get priority over limb-threatening diseases and have to be dealt with first when considering surgery.

Authors prefer to treat the associated hydrocephalus in the same sitting. Associated syrinx may be punctured and drained or left untouched, as it is not a worry once the primary pathology has been taken care of. Authors generally have never had to deal with associated Chiari, which usually resolves once MMC has been repaired. Anything that is life-threatening for the patient has to be corrected first. For instance, in OEIS complex, consisting of omphalocele, exstrophy of the cloaca, imperforate anus, and spinal defects, as the first three defects are life-threatening, they need to be treated on a priority basis and neurosurgery takes a back seat.[60]

Postoperative complications like CSF leak, pseudomeningocele, and meningitis should be watched for. Prolonged surgery at multiple sites can have various complications like severe blood loss and hypothermia, especially in children, which eventually leads to postoperative morbidity.

Conclusion

Complex SCM is an important cliniconeuroradiological presentation of spinal dysraphisms. There is increasing mention of this in literature, because of appropriate screening methodology. It has opened up debates on the underlying embryological mechanisms and therefore requires experimental studies. The most important step in management is to be aware of its existence and look for it. MRI forms an important tool in our toolbox to pinpoint the associated anomalies and deal with them appropriately. The surgical principles remain the same; however, the risk of complications is a little higher with complex forms of dysraphism. These patients also require a close long-term follow-up to look for new onset neurological deficits.

References

1. Tortori-Donati P, Rossi A, Cama A. Spinal dysraphism: a review of neuroradiological features with embryological correlations and proposal for a new classification. Neuroradiology 2000;42(7): 471–491
2. Dias MS, Walker ML. The embryogenesis of complex dysraphic malformations: a disorder of gastrulation? Pediatr Neurosurg 1992;18(5–6):229–253
3. Kumar R, Bansal KK, Chhabra DK. Occurrence of split cord malformation in meningomyelocele: complex spina bifida. Pediatr Neurosurg 2002;36(3):119–127
4. Kumar R, Singh V, Singh SN. Split cord malformation in children undergoing neurological intervention in India: a descriptive study. J Pediatr Neurol 2004;2:21–27
5. Garg K, Kumar R. Complex split cord malformation type 1 with multiple lipomas involving the split cord. Pediatr Neurosurg 2013;49(2):121–123
6. Salunke P, Futane SS, Aggarwal A. Split cord malformation Type II with twin dorsal lipomas. J Neurosurg Pediatr 2012;9(6):627–629
7. Gök A, Bayram M, Coşkun Y, Ozsaraç C. Unusual malformations in occult spinal dysraphism. Turk J Pediatr 1995;37(4):391–397
8. Piegger J, Gruber H, Fritsch H. Case report: human neonatus with spina bifida, clubfoot, situs inversus totalis and cerebral deformities: sequence or accident? Ann Anat 2000;182(6):577–581

9. Garg K, Kumar R. Complex spinal dysraphism with multiple anomalies. Pediatr Neurosurg 2013; 49(2):126–128

10. Buyukkaya A, Özel MA, Buyukkaya R, Onbas Ö. Complex split cord malformation. Spine J 2015;15(7): 1693–1694

11. Patnaik A, Mahapatra AK. Complex forms of spinal dysraphism. Childs Nerv Syst 2013;29(9): 1527–1532

12. Sewell MJ, Chiu YE, Drolet BA, Drolet BA. Neural tube dysraphism: review of cutaneous markers and imaging. Pediatr Dermatol 2015;32(2):161–170

13. Pang D, Dias MS, Ahab-Barmada M. Split cord malformation: Part I: A unified theory of embryogenesis for double spinal cord malformations. Neurosurgery 1992;31(3):451–480

14. Forrester MB, Merz RD. Descriptive epidemiology of lipomyelomeningocele, Hawaii, 1986–2001. Birth Defects Res A Clin Mol Teratol 2004;70(12):953–956

15. Dhandapani S, Srinivasan A. Contiguous triple spinal dysraphism associated with Chiari malformation Type II and hydrocephalus: an embryological conundrum between the unified theory of Pang and the unified theory of McLone. J Neurosurg Pediatr 2016;17(1):103–106

16. Dhandapani S, Mehta VS, Sharma BS. "Horseshoe cord terminus" sans filum around a bone spur: a rare composite of faulty gastrulation with agenesis of secondary neurulation: case report. J Neurosurg Pediatr 2013;12(4):411–413

17. Kapoor A, Dhandapani S, Singh P. The triad of holocord syringomyelia, Chiari malformation and tethered cord: amelioration with simple detethering—a case for revisiting traction hypothesis? Neurol India 2014;62(6):708–709

18. McLone DG, Knepper PA. The cause of Chiari II malformation: a unified theory. Pediatr Neurosci 1989;15(1):1–12

19. Solanki GA, Evans J, Copp A, Thompson DN. Multiple coexistent dysraphic pathologies. Childs Nerv Syst 2003;19(5-6):376–379

20. Srinivas D, Sharma BS, Mahapatra AK. Triple neural tube defect and the multisite closure theory for neural tube defects: is there an additional site? Case report. J Neurosurg Pediatr 2008;1(2):160–163

21. Tekkök IH. Triple neural tube defect—cranium bifidum with rostral and caudal spina bifida—live evidence of multi-site closure of the neural tube in humans. Childs Nerv Syst 2005;21(4):331–335

22. Ross JS, Brant-Zawadzki M, Moore KR, Crim J, Chen MZ, Katzman GL. Diagnostic Imaging: Spine. 1st ed. Altona: Amirsys Inc; 2004

23. Ikenouchi J, Uwabe C, Nakatsu T, Hirose M, Shiota K. Embryonic hydromyelia: cystic dilatation of the lumbosacral neural tube in human embryos. Acta Neuropathol 2002;103(3):248–254

24. Tortori-Donati P, Rossi A, Biancheri R, Cama A. Magnetic resonance imaging of spinal dysraphism. Top Magn Reson Imaging 2001;12(6):375–409

25. Gardner WJ. Hypothesis; overdistention of the neural tube may cause anomalies of non-neural organs. Teratology 1980;22(2):229–238

26. Kumar R, Singh SN, Bansal KK, Singh V. Comparative study of complex spina bifida and split cord malformation. Indian J Pediatr 2005;72(2):109–115

27. Ozturk E, Sonmez G, Mutlu H, et al. Split-cord malformation and accompanying anomalies. J Neuroradiol 2008;35(3):150–156

28. Higashida T, Sasano M, Sato H, Sekido K, Ito S. Myelomeningocele associated with split cord malformation type I -three case reports-. Neurol Med Chir (Tokyo) 2010;50(5):426–430

29. Akiyama K, Nishiyama K, Yoshimura J, Mori H, Fujii Y. A case of split cord malformation associated with myeloschisis. Childs Nerv Syst 2007;23(5):577–580

30. Yamanaka T, Hashimoto N, Sasajima H, Mineura K. A case of diastematomyelia associated with myeloschisis in a hemicord. Pediatr Neurosurg 2001;35(5):253–256

31. Jans L, Vlummens P, Van Damme S, Verstraete K, Abernethy L. Hemimyelomeningocele: a rare and complex spinal dysraphism. JBR-BTR 2008;91(5):198–199

32. Rowley VB, Johnson AJ. Lumbar split cord malformation with lateral hemimyelomeningocele and associated Chiari II malformation and other visceral and osseous anomalies: a case report. J Comput Assist Tomogr 2009;33(6):923–926

33. Singh N, Singh DK, Kumar R. Diastematomyelia with hemimyelomeningocele: an exceptional and complex spinal dysraphism. J Pediatr Neurosci 2015;10(3):237–239

34. Parmar H, Patkar D, Shah J, Maheshwari M. Diastematomyelia with terminal lipomyelocystocele arising from one hemicord: case report. Clin Imaging 2003;27(1):41–43

35. Khandelwal A, Tandon V, Mahapatra AK. An unusual case of 4 level spinal dysraphism: Multiple composite type 1 and type 2 split cord malformation, dorsal myelocystocele and hydrocephalous. J Pediatr Neurosci 2011;6(1):58–61

36. Emmez H, Tokgöz N, Dogulu F, Yilmaz MB, Kale A, Baykaner MK. Seven distinct coexistent cranial and spinal anomalies. Pediatr Neurosurg 2006;42(5):316–319

37. Avcu S, Köseoğlu MN, Bulut MD, Ozen O, Unal O. The association of tethered cord, syringomyelia, diastometamyelia, spinal epidermoid, spinal lipoma and dermal sinus tract in a child. JBR-BTR 2010;93(6):305–307

38. Maiti TK, Bhat DI, Devi BI, Sampath S, Mahadevan A, Shankar SK. Teratoma in split cord malformation: an unusual association: a report of two cases with a review of the literature. Pediatr Neurosurg 2010;46(3):238–241

39. Naik V, Mahapatra AK, Gupta C, Suri V. Complex split cord malformation with mediastinal extension of a teratoma and simultaneous ventral and dorsal bony spur splitting the cord. Pediatr Neurosurg 2010;46(5):368–372

40. Ugarte N, Gonzalez-Crussi F, Sotelo-Avila C. Diastematomyelia associated with teratomas. Report of two cases. J Neurosurg 1980;53(5):720–725

41. Harwood-Nash DC, McHugh K. Diastematomyelia in 172 children: the impact of modern neuroradiology. Pediatr Neurosurg 1990-1991;16(4-5):247–251

42. Pang D. Split cord malformation: Part II: Clinical syndrome. Neurosurgery 1992;31(3):481–500

43. Erşahin Y, Mutluer S, Kocaman S, Demirtaş E. Split spinal cord malformations in children. J Neurosurg 1998;88(1):57–65

44. Ailawadhi P, Mahapatra AK. An unusual case of spinal dysraphism with four splits including three posterior spurs. Pediatr Neurosurg 2011;47(5):372–375

45. Singh PK, Khandelwal A, Singh A, Ailawadhi P, Gupta D, Mahapatra AK. Long-segment type 1 split cord malformation with two-level split cord malformation and a single dural sac at the lower split. Pediatr Neurosurg 2011;47(3):227–229

46. Vaishya S, Kumarjain P. Split cord malformation: three unusual cases of composite split cord malformation. Childs Nerv Syst 2001;17(9):528–530

47. Akay KM, Izci Y, Baysefer A, Timurkaynak E. Composite type of split cord malformation: two different types at three different levels: case report. J Neurosurg 2005; 102(4, Suppl):436–438

48. Jarmundowicz W, Tabakow P, Markowska-Woyciechowska A. Composite split cord malformation coexisting with spinal cord teratoma—case report and review of the literature. Folia Neuropathol 2004;42(1):55–57

49. Dwarakanath S, Suri A, Garg A, Mahapatra AK, Mehta VS. Adult complex spinal dysraphism with situs inversus totalis: a rare association and review. Spine 2005;30(8):E225–E228

50. Tubbs RS, Wellons JC III, Oakes WJ. Split cord malformation and situs inversus totalis: case report and review of the literature. Childs Nerv Syst 2005;21(2):161–164

51. Karrer FM, Flannery AM, Nelson MD, McLone DG, Raffensperger JG. Anorectal malformations: evaluation of associated spinal dysraphic syndromes. J Pediatr Surg 1988;23(1):45–48

52. Neel N, Tarabay MS. Omphalocele, exstrophy of cloaca, imperforate anus, and spinal defect complex, multiple major reconstructive surgeries needed. Urol Ann 2018;10(1):118–121

53. Shieh C, Lam CH. A lateral cervical lipomyelomeningocele associated with diplomyelia. Pediatr Neurosurg 2006;42(6):399–403

54. Ansari S, Nejat F, Yazdani S, Dadmehr M. Split cord malformation associated with myelomeningocele. J Neurosurg 2007;107(4, Suppl):281–285

55. Kumar R, Singh SN, Bansal KK, Singh V. Comparative study of complex spina bifida and split cord malformation. Indian J Pediatr 2005;72(2):109–115

56. Yoshioka F, Shimokawa S, Koguchi M, et al. Curved planar reformation for the evaluation of hydromyelia in patients with scoliosis associated with spinal dysraphism. Spine 2018;43(3):E177–E184

57. Rauzzino MJ, Tubbs RS, Alexander E III, Grabb PA, Oakes WJ. Spinal neurenteric cysts and their relation to more common aspects of occult spinal dysraphism. Neurosurg Focus 2001;10(1):e2

58. Chern JJ, Kirkman JL, Shannon CN, et al. Use of lumbar ultrasonography to detect occult spinal dysraphism. J Neurosurg Pediatr 2012;9(3):274–279

59. Ausili E, Maresca G, Massimi L, Morgante L, Romagnoli C, Rendeli C. Occult spinal dysraphisms in newborns with skin markers: role of ultrasonography and magnetic resonance imaging. Childs Nerv Syst 2018;34(2):285–291

60. Morioka T, Hashiguchi K, Yoshida F, et al. Neurosurgical management of occult spinal dysraphism associated with OEIS complex. Childs Nerv Syst 2008;24(6):723–729

Prophylactic Surgery in Split Cord Malformations

Vivek Tandon, Skanda Moorthy, and Ashok K. Mahapatra

Table of Contents

■ Introduction 113

■ Clinical Presentation 113

■ Investigations 114

■ Treatment 114

■ Outcome 115

Prophylactic Surgery in Split Cord Malformations

Vivek Tandon, Skanda Moorthy, and Ashok K. Mahapatra

Introduction

Split cord malformations (SCMs) are a rare type of spinal dysraphism, and they are usually associated with low-lying tethered cords. SCMs constitute about one-third of spinal dysraphisms.[1] Type I SCM has two hemicords in two separate dural sacs split by a bony spur present over variable spinal segments, and Type II has both the hemicords in the same dural sac and are split by a membranous septum. Type I SCMs have four subtypes, depending upon the location of the bony spur.[2] The most common location of SCM is dorsal and lumbar spine, and rarely can they be encountered in cervical or sacral areas.[3] In a newborn, conus ends at L3 level and as the child grows due to disproportionate growth of cord and vertebral segments, there is ascent of the cord till its final adult level of L1. SCM and low-lying tethered cord may be linked with a variety of other anomalies like conus lipoma, myelomeningocele, lipomeningomyelocele, dermal sinus tract, or meningocele.

As children with these malformations may be completely asymptomatic, controversy exists regarding prophylactic surgery in these patients. Low-lying cord can often be associated with scoliosis both congenital as well as secondary to weakness of paraspinous muscles. Prophylactic detethering before scoliosis correction is a preferred option in case of a low-lying cord.[4-6] Prophylactic detethering increases the mobility of the cord inside the vertebral column; hence, decreasing the chances of damage during corrective surgery. However, there are opinions against the same on the basis that prophylactic surgery does not improve the neurological status. In contrast, it may cause deterioration, and is also associated with other neurosurgical complications like cerebrospinal fluid (CSF) leak, infection and neurological deterioration.[7,8] Other factors against detethering include loss of posterior bony elements, which may contribute to further osseous defects and potential for regrowth of the spur.[9,10] The option of prophylactic surgery with all its pros and cons should be discussed with the patients, and in this chapter we present our view, based on existing literature and our vast experience.

Clinical Presentation

Most of these patients present in early childhood either due to neurocutaneous stigmata or development of neurological deficits and deformity; however, there are incidents of patients presenting in the adulthood either due to back pain, neurological symptoms, or they may be completely asymptomatic. Associated tethering of the cord leads to limited cord movement and stretching while flexion and extension of back. This chronic stretching of the cord leads to ischemic insult to the cord and results in neurological symptoms. Various presenting clinical features include hypertrichosis in the back, dermal sinus, chronic back pain, numbness in the foot, weakness of lower limbs, bladder bowel incontinence, and scoliosis which may occur due to weakness of paraspinal muscles on either side.[11,12]

Occasionally, physicians diagnose patients incidentally. These patients do not have neurological symptoms but are diagnosed due to presence of cutaneous stigmata, scoliosis, or radiological screening for any other cause.

Investigations

MRI is the investigative modality of choice; contrast should be used when a dermoid or teratoma is suspected on initial imaging. On MRI imaging, presence of two hemicords separated by a bony septum in two separate dural sheaths is diagnostic of Type I SCM, while a membranous septa separating the two hemicords in a single dural sheath is suggestive of Type II SCM. In about 50% of the cases, they occur at L1–L3 levels, and in about 25%, they occur at D7–D12 levels; in the rest 25% cases, they may occur at a higher level. Associated findings include scoliosis or other anomalies like lipomyelomeningocele and dermal sinus tract. Normal filum terminale is less than 2 mm thick. A thick fatty filum with lower than usual cord ending level (below L2) is a common finding in these cases (**Fig. 11.1**).

Other useful investigations include CT scan to better delineate the bony spur, urodynamic studies for bladder function, and ultrasound abdomen to study the kidneys, ureter, bladder and postvoid urine residue.

All patients must also undergo routine hematological investigations, urine routine microscopy, and renal function tests. Urine culture and sensitivity is to be done in symptomatic cases or where urine routine microscopy is suggestive of infection.

Treatment

SCM with low-lying cord when detected in childhood should be treated as early as possible. Detethering of the low-lying cord by excising the bony spur or membranous septa and cutting the tethered and fatty filum would increase the mobility of the cord inside the dural sac and prevent the development of chronic stretch-related neurological deficits.[13–15] Considering that the established neurological deficits

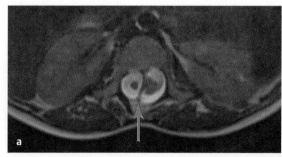
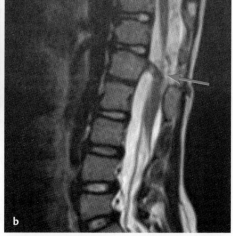

Fig. 11.1 (a) T2WI showing Type I SCM. **(b)** T2WI sagittal image, demonstrating low-lying cord with bony spur.

are usually irreversible, surgical option should be considered in children with SCM, even when they are asymptomatic.

However, if low-lying cord is incidentally diagnosed in adults, then these patients should be thoroughly evaluated clinically for subtle signs of neurological and urological deficits. In presence of subtle deficits, option of surgery should be given. If such patients are only having axial backache, then treatment remains controversial. Many studies suggest conservative follow up is as good as surgery.[16] Low backache may persist even after the detethering operation, and 5 to 50% patients may have retethering and may need reoperation (**Table 11.1**).[13,17–19]

Conventionally, detethering operation prior to scoliosis correction surgery is considered. Detethering increases the mobility of the cord and decreases the chances of damage in scoliosis corrective surgery. However, this viewpoint has been challenged by Shen et al, who have corrected scoliosis without detethering and have reported comparable results.[20]

Surgical treatment includes a small midline linear incision at L5–S1 level, followed by laminectomy or interlaminar approach to reach the thecal sac. Vertical dural incision is given nerve roots and thick filum identified. Filum terminale is identified as white glistening structure. After ensuring that the filum is free of nerve roots all around, it should be coagulated. It should be made sure that proximal part of the filum, and hence the cord, is free of any attachments which prevent its free motion. In case of type I SCM, another incision should be made at the level of bony spur. After laminectomy, bony spur should be identified, which in majority of the cases is attached anteriorly to the vertebral body and running posteriorly and, occasionally, may be attached posteriorly to the posterior part of lamina.[21,22] After excision of the bony spur, dural opening should be made, starting at the normal cord and should be extended on to the hemicords on both the sacs. Aberrant nerves, arachnoid adhesions, and any other structures tethering the cord should be coagulated and excised to free the cord.

Split cord should be explored first followed by filum detethering to prevent cord damage due to ascent of cord.

Outcome

There is halt in the progress of neurological deterioration in majority of patients, while some patients (10–15%) may have deterioration in the neurological status as a complication of surgical intervention. In less than 10% cases, retethering and regrowth of the bony spur have been described.[23] Other complications like infection and CSF leak have been reported in 7 to 31% of patients.[7,8]

Table 11.1 Management plan for SCMs with low-lying cord in different age groups

Age group	Clinical condition	Treatment
Children	Asymptomatic	Surgery
	Symptomatic	
Adults	Asymptomatic, backache	Surgery/conservative
	Neurological deficits, scoliosis requiring correction	Surgery

Abbreviation: SCMs, split cord malformations.

References

1. Kumar R, Singh V, Singh SN. Split cord malformation in children undergoing neurological intervention in India: a descriptive study. J Pediatr Neurol 2004;2:21–27
2. Mahapatra AK, Gupta DK. Split cord malformations: a clinical study of 254 patients and a proposal for a new clinical-imaging classification. J Neurosurg 2005; 103(6, Suppl):531–536
3. Mahapatra AK. Split cord malformation: a study of 300 cases at AIIMS 1990–2006. J Pediatr Neurosci 2011;6(Suppl 1):S41–S45
4. Proctor MR, Scott RM. Long-term outcome for patients with split cord malformation. Neurosurg Focus 2001;10(1):e5
5. Frerebeau P, Dimeglio A, Gras M, Harbi H. Diastematomyelia: report of 21 cases surgically treated by a neurosurgical and orthopedic team. Childs Brain 1983;10(5):328–339
6. Goldberg C, Fenelon G, Blake NS, Dowling F, Regan BF. Diastematomyelia: a critical review of the natural history and treatment. Spine 1984;9(4):367–372
7. Ayvaz M, Alanay A, Yazici M, Acaroglu E, Akalan N, Aksoy C. Safety and efficacy of posterior instrumentation for patients with congenital scoliosis and spinal dysraphism. J Pediatr Orthop 2007;27(4):380–386
8. Sinha S, Agarwal D, Mahapatra AK. Split cord malformations: an experience of 203 cases. Childs Nerv Syst 2006;22(1):3–7
9. Gupta DK, Ahmed S, Garg K, Mahapatra AK. Regrowth of septal spur in split cord malformation. Pediatr Neurosurg 2010;46(3):242–244
10. Pang D, Parrish RG. Regrowth of diastematomyelic bone spur after extradural resection. Case report. J Neurosurg 1983;59(5):887–890
11. Frainey BT, Yerkes EB, Menon VS, et al. Predictors of urinary continence following tethered cord release in children with occult spinal dysraphism. J Pediatr Urol 2014;10(4):627–633
12. Yener S, Thomas DT, Hicdonmez T, et al. The effect of untethering on urologic symptoms and urodynamic parameters in children with primary tethered cord syndrome. Urology 2015;85(1): 221–226
13. Thuy M, Chaseling R, Fowler A. Spinal cord detethering procedures in children: a 5 year retrospective cohort study of the early post-operative course. J Clin Neurosci 2015;22(5):838–842
14. Gharedaghi M, Samini F, Mashhadinejad H, Khajavi M, Samini M. Orthopedic lesions in tethered cord syndrome: the importance of early diagnosis and treatment on patient outcome. Arch Bone Jt Surg 2014;2(2):93–97
15. Stavrinou P, Kunz M, Lehner M, et al. Children with tethered cord syndrome of different etiology benefit from microsurgery: a single institution experience. Childs Nerv Syst 2011;27(5):803–810
16. Steinbok P, MacNeily AE, Hengel AR, et al. Filum section for urinary incontinence in children with occult tethered cord syndrome: a randomized, controlled pilot study. J Urol 2016;195(4 Pt 2): 1183–1188
17. Akay KM, Izci Y, Baysefer A, Timurkaynak E. Split cord malformation in adults. Neurosurg Rev 2004;27(2):99–105
18. Vassilyadi M, Tataryn Z, Merziotis M. Retethering in children after sectioning of the filum terminale. Pediatr Neurosurg 2012;48(6):335–341
19. Mehta VA, Bettegowda C, Ahmadi SA, et al. Spinal cord tethering following myelomeningocele repair. J Neurosurg Pediatr 2010;6(5):498–505
20. Shen J, Zhang J, Feng F, Wang Y, Qiu G, Li Z. Corrective surgery for congenital scoliosis associated with split cord malformation: it may be safe to leave diastematomyelia untreated in patients with intact or stable neurological status. J Bone Joint Surg Am 2016;98(11):926–936

21. Akay KM, Izci Y, Baysefer A. Dorsal bony septum: a split cord malformation variant. Pediatr Neurosurg 2002;36(5):225–228

22. Chandra PS, Kamal R, Mahapatra AK. An unusual case of dorsally situated bony spur in a lumbar split cord malformation. Pediatr Neurosurg 1999;31(1):49–52

23. Feng F, Shen J, Zhang J, et al. Clinical outcomes of different surgical strategy for patients with congenital scoliosis and type 1 split cord malformation. Spine 2016;41(16):1310–1316

Protocol for Management of Split Cord Malformations

Vivek Tandon, Harish Chandrappa, and Ashok K. Mahapatra

Table of Contents

■ Introduction 121

■ Clinical Presentation.. 121

■ Classification 121

■ Investigations... 122

■ Management... 124

■ Role of Neuromonitoring....................................... 129

■ Postoperative Care 129

■ Complications, Prevention, and
   Their Management 129

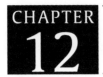
CHAPTER 12

Protocol for Management of Split Cord Malformations

Vivek Tandon, Harish Chandrappa, and Ashok K. Mahapatra

Introduction

Split cord malformations (SCMs), being occult spinal dysraphisms, are rare congenital anomalies of the spinal cord. With advent of MRI and rising awareness of physicians, pediatricians and orthopedicians, an increasing number of asymptomatic or occult malformations are being diagnosed and referred to the neurosurgeons.

Clinical Presentation

Patients may present with various symptomatology of either deformity of back, limb deformity or progressive neurological deficits including tethered cord syndrome.[1,2,3,4,5]

Patients may also be asymptomatic, with only cutaneous stigmata.[2,6]

Adults may present only with backache (**Box 12.1**).[7]

Classification

Pang classified the SCM into type I and II.[1] Type I was further classified into four types by Gupta and Mahapatra, based on the relation of the bony spur to the cord and risk of operative injury to the cord and, in turn, the risk of postoperative neurological deficits (**Table 12.1**).[2]

Box 12.1 Various symptoms/signs of SCM

- Backache
- Progressive neurological deficits
- Orthopedic syndrome
- Urinary disturbances
- Sensory disturbances
- Asymptomatic:
  - ◇ Cutaneous stigmata
  - ◇ Hypertrichosis/Faun's tail
  - ◇ Capillary hemangioma
  - ◇ Subcutaneous lipoma
  - ◇ Skin tags
  - ◇ Dermal sinus
  - ◇ Sacral dimple

Table 12.1 Classification of SCM

SCM type	Anatomic	Radiographic	Location
I	• Two hemicords in two dural sleeves separated by a midline bony spur. • Hypertrophic laminae are often fused to adjacent levels.	• MRI—Two hemicords with two separate dural sleeves (subarachnoid space) separated by a bony spur (**Fig. 12.1a**). • CT—Bony spur with intersegmental fusion and spina bifida.	Typically lumbar.
II	Two hemicords in a single dural sleeve. Hemicords are separated and tethered by a fibrous band attached to the dura.	Two hemicords with a single subarachnoid space on T2W MRI, with or without a fibrous septum (**Fig. 12.1b**).	May occur anywhere along the spinal axis.

Abbreviation: SCM, split cord malformation.

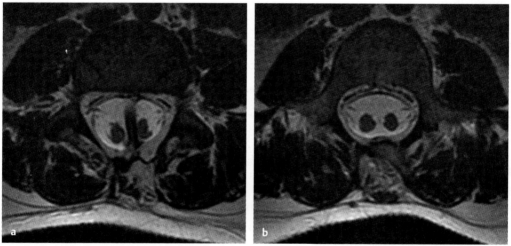

Fig. 12.1 (a) Type I split cord malformations (SCM)—T2W MRI axial section, showing two hemicords enclosed in two separate subarachnoid space, with an hypointense bony spur. **(b)** Type II SCM—Two hemicords enclosed in a single subarachnoid space.

Type I could be further classified as follows (see also **Fig. 3.5** in Chapter 3):

- **Type Ia:** Bony spur in the center with equally duplicated cord above and below the spur.
- **Type Ib:** Bony spur at the superior pole with no space above and a large duplicated cord lower down.
- **Type Ic:** Bony spur at the lower pole with a large duplicated cord above.
- **Type Id:** Bony spur straddling the bifurcation with no space above or below the spur.

Investigations

X-ray: May detect the occult spina bifida, abnormal curvature of the spine. Also, helps in identification of bony landmarks, and a preoperative Marker X-ray may be used to reduce operative time and radiation exposure in the operating room (OR).[2,5]

MRI: It is the most common and usually the first investigation of choice for the diagnosis of SCMs. The typical feature is the presence of two hemicords, duplicated or in a single dural sheath as seen on T1W and T2W images, respectively. Presence of a bony spur may also be visualized.

Also, MRI can show other tethering elements like lipoma, fatty filum, dermal sinus, neuroenteric cyst, or dermoid. Because multiple tethering elements may be present, all patients with suspected spinal dysraphism and patients with scoliosis should get an axial MRI of whole spine to rule out any split or tethering elements elsewhere[3] (**Fig. 12.2**).

Brain imaging is warranted only when clinical suspicion of hydrocephalus or of any other congenital anomaly is present or there is an associated Chiari malformation on the spine MRI.

CT scan: CT is most useful in cases of SCM I to delineate the bony spur and plan surgery. It may also be helpful in detecting associated vertebral segmentation anomalies like hemivertebra, bifid vertebra, bifid laminae and Klippel–Feil syndrome, and planning deformity correction.

Ultrasonography (USG): USG is helpful in looking for dilated urinary bladder, postvoid residue, and hydroureteronephrosis. Also, associated renal and genitourinary malformations may be identified.

Urodynamic studies (UDS): Urinary incontinence being one of the common problems, early detection and treatment of the urological disorder is of utmost importance to prevent secondary damage. UDS is important for diagnosis, follow-up, and prognostication of the patient.[8,9]

Common abnormalities noted are overactive bladder, reduced capacity, postvoid residue, reduced compliance, underactive bladder, and dyssynergia. These changes need to be identified early and need correction before upper tract is damaged or chronic kidney disease sets in.

Renal function tests: Renal dysfunction, although a late feature, is vital to be recognized, and due precautions, in the form of avoiding nephrotoxic drugs and catheterization or clean intermittent catheterization (CIC), need to be taken to avoid further injury.

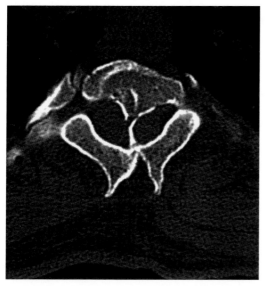

Fig. 12.2 Axial section of dorsal spine, showing bifid spinous process and complete bony spur—features of split cord malformations (SCM) type I.

Urine microscopy and cultures: To rule out active urinary tract infections preoperatively.

Muscle charting: Muscle power charting of each muscle or muscle group is a useful adjunct for documentation, future references, and comparisons in the postoperative period and follow-up of the patient.

Management

■ Indications

All children with both Type I or II SCM should be operated as it has been observed that risk of progressive neurological deterioration is very high up to 85%, due to tethering of the ascending cord in growing children, as compared to a reasonably low risk involved in surgery.

All patients of scoliosis, and any other spinal dysraphisms, should undergo evaluation for SCM. If present, these need to be addressed prior to or in the same setting, as the deformity correction is considered in case of scoliosis.

In adults, patients with progressive neurological deficits, radiculopathy or back pain warrant surgery. Evidence is less compelling, with respect to asymptomatic adults with SCM. However, these patients may have sudden neurological worsening after trivial trauma or even strenuous exercises. Hence, as a principle of good practice, surgery may be offered to adult patients who are prone to trauma or lead an active lifestyle, while observing old patients with medical comorbid illness and having sedentary lifestyle.

All patients need to undergo exploration of all tethering elements and detethering. In case of SCM I, bony spur needs to be resected with unification of dural sac and detethering of the conus by cutting the filum, especially when low lying.

In type II SCM, fibrous septae dividing the two hemicords or the adhesive bands may be thin and not appreciable on imaging. However, these should be explored, any fibrous septae need to be removed, and the bands be divided. Even the ventral aspect of the cord needs exploration for the same.

Any other tethering elements like lipoma, neuroenteric cyst, myelomeningocele manqué, dermal sinus tracts, or dermoids also need to be addressed in the same setting.[2,4,10] See **Flowchart 12.1** for algorithm for management of SCM.

■ Preoperative Preparation

Multidisciplinary approach involving neurosurgeons, pediatric surgeons, pediatricians, plastic surgeons, and anesthesiologists is of prime importance in the management of these patients. Associated anomalies, especially anorectal malformations or genitourinary tract, should be addressed, if possible, in the same setting.

Care should be taken to identify the renal function abnormalities and avoid nephrotoxic drugs including anesthetic agents in the perioperative period.

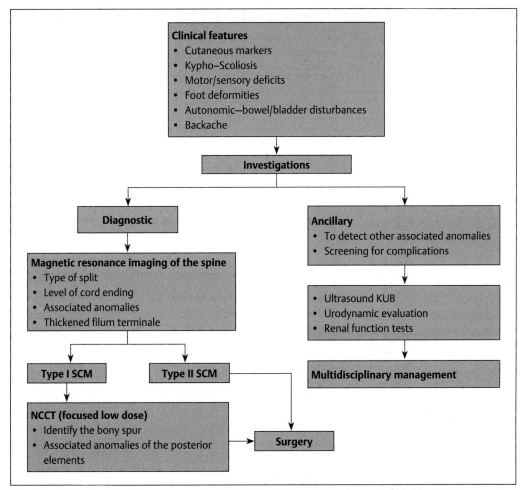

Flowchart 12.1 Algorithm for management of SCM. Abbreviations: KUB, kidney ureter bladder; NCCT, noncontrast computed tomography scan; SCM, split cord malformation.

■ Surgical Procedure

Position

Patients are put in prone position after induction, with appropriate padding of the pressure points, and care is taken to prevent hypothermia.

Identification of the Right Level

Level is to be confirmed with C-arm or preoperative marker X-ray, as often the cutaneous stigmata may not exactly correspond to the level of split. Midline incision is planned, so as to span at least two levels above and below the split. Exposure of the said level, identification of normal anatomy, and dissection from normal to the morbid anatomy is of crucial importance. The bony septum is extradural and is usually hidden by the neural arches. Wider spinal canal at the level of the split, associated hypertrophic neural arches, or spinous processes may help in identification of the level. Associated bony anomalies adjacent to the septum-like bifid spinous processes, bifid laminae, abnormal fusion anomalies, eccentric laminae, or exostoses are also of localizing value and need to be studied on preoperative imaging.

Exposure

Adequate exposure of at least one level above and below the identified split levels should be done, dissecting subperiosteally.

From here, surgery for Type I and II SCM will differ.

Surgery for Type I SCM

Lamiectomy and Isolation of Spur

Laminectomy should extend one level above and below the split. Laminectomy may be done with high-speed drill or ronguers in a piecemeal manner, so as to isolate a small island attached to the bony spur. The spur can now be visualized all around, and the dura can be dissected away from it under vision. Due care needs to be taken to not exert lateral pressure on the septum, as now its dorsolateral supports have been removed and may move freely and compress upon the hemicord on the opposite side.

Most bony septum have broad dorsal attachment and thin flimsy ventral attachment to the vertebral body, and may be easily avulse from the dural cleft, taking due care not to press upon the hemicords, especially on the inferior aspect. When the ventral attachment is stout and bony, it needs to be taken away with either ronguers or careful drilling under continuous copious irrigation, so as to avoid thermal injury. End point of the drilling is when it becomes flush with the vertebral body. The spur is vascular and may have an embedded central artery, which bleeds profusely on resection and may be controlled by bone wax.

As per the subclassification of Type I SCM, type Ia being the most common type, they have wide space on either side of the bony spur for dissection and margin for drilling.

Type Ib have bony spur at the superior end of the split and widely separate hemicords below. In these, dissection and drilling from inferior end is warranted, as there is a narrow space above the septum and any handling in this already compromised cord may lead to significant neurological deficits.

Type Ic have spur at the lower aspect of the split and need to be approached from superior end.

Type Id is characterized by bony spur snugly fitting into the split and practically no space on either side of the cord. Risk of neurological deterioration is high in these patients. However, these may be approached from superior aspect, as the ascending cord tends to tightly abut the lower end of the spur. Alternatively, the central core of the spur may be addressed first to make it eggshell-like and then dissected off the dura centrally and removed in a piecemeal manner (**Fig. 12.3**).

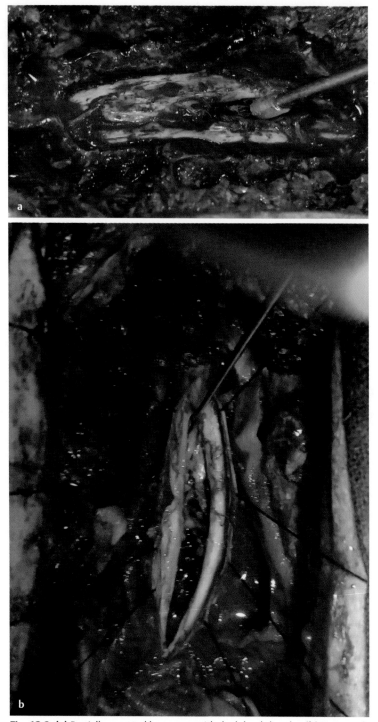

Fig. 12.3 (a) Partially resected bony spur with dual dural sheaths. **(b)** Twin cords adjacent to resected bony spur and dural hitch sutures, before reconstruction of single dural sheath.

Unification of Dural Sacs

The duramater is now opened around the midline cleft to isolate this median dural sleeve. The medial aspect of the hemicords may be adherent to the dural sleeve, which needs to be sharply divided. The dorsomedial nerve roots spanning from the dorsomedial aspect of the hemicord and ending at the dural sleeve are nonfunctional and are to be divided before excision of the sleeve, so as to prevent undue traction over the cords. As already mentioned, inferior end of the split is often tightly abutting the dural sleeve, as the cord is ascending; hence, the superior end is relatively safe to start the excision of dural sleeve. It needs to be coagulated to prevent bleeding from the retracted dural ends and cut flush with the ventral dura. Now, the median cleft should be examined for any residual stump of the spur and drilled flush, if any.

Posterior edges of dura is closed to make it a single dural sac. Dura closure needs to be meticulous with or without a dural patch, using locally available thoracolumbar fascia. Some surgeons may prefer artificial dural substitutes. Suture material is again a matter of surgeon's choice. Previously 4–0 PDS or vicryl were widely used, although with time it is observed that smaller sutures with smaller needles are less traumatic to the dura and help in better closure, avoiding mini-needle holes along the suture line. Hence, some may prefer 6–0 and some even 10–0 suture materials like prolene or nylon.

Closure of ventral dura is unnecessary, as there are usually adhesions between the ventral dura and the posterior longitudinal ligament, preventing cerebrospinal fluid (CSF) leak. Also, it may be detrimental, as ventral suture line may act as a future tethering point.

Other Intradural Pathologies

Associated anomalies like lipoma, demoid, or lipomeningocele need to be addressed, and cord should be detethered from these tethering structures.

Surgery for Type II SCM

Laminectomy/Laminotomy

Laminae may be drilled on either sides and then lifted as a hinge, which can be resutured at the end in small children with malleable bony elements. In older children and adults, either a focused single or 2 level laminectomy/hemilaminectomy is done, or longer laminotomy may be done, which may be refixed with miniplate and screws at the end of the procedure.

Division of the Septum

Dura opened in midline and the dividing septum identified. They can be of the following types:

- **Complete fibrous septum:** Analogous to spur in type I, it spans whole of the sac dorsoventrally. It is the least common type.
- **Pure ventral septum:** Not readily visible and has to be looked for by rotating the hemicords.
- **Pure dorsal septum:** Most common.

Filum Terminale Transection

Filum terminale should be cut irrespective of the conus level in all cases of SCM. This can be done with extension of the same incision for exploration of split if lower down or one may give a fresh incision below the level of conus, commonly L5–S1 interspace.

Filum can be identified by its pale and shiny surface, without any trabeculations, having a single tortuous vessel running ventrally, unlike the nerve roots which are dull, yellowish, with trabeculations and with a mesh network of capillaries over them. Filum should be freed from all the nerve roots all around and then thoroughly coagulated and divided in small cuts, so that any bleed can be coagulated. The proximal end may be seen to retract and ascend once divided, and if any residual vessel may continue to bleed into the thecal sac.

Role of Neuromonitoring

Due to proximity of the cord or the conus to the bony spur or the fibrous septa, it involves a high risk of neurological deterioration while manipulating them. Motor-evoked potentials (MEP), somatosensory-evoked potentials (SSEP), and sphincter functions may be used to monitor the function, so that fall in amplitude of the responses may be recorded, last surgical step may be stopped and reversed if possible, and appropriate change in the surgical technique is adapted to reduce the damage.[11] Responses obtained from anal sphincter also corroborate with bladder function, as both are supplied by the nervi erigentes S2–S5.[11] Also, direct stimulation of the nerve roots may be done whenever required to identify the filum terminale while detethering.

Postoperative Care

- It is recommended to nurse the children in prone position with head down to prevent CSF leak.
- Sedation may be necessary to calm the children, prevent them from wiggling and pulling at the incision, and also to prevent cry, and Valsalva maneuver, which may hamper healing and cause CSF leak.
- Some urinary retention may be seen commonly in the postop period, which is mostly transient and may last for up to a few months. A catheter is left in situ till the first postop day, when the child is encouraged to mobilize, and trail of catheter removal may be given. If there is problem in micturition or retention occurs, a trial of detrusor training over the next few days to a week through frequent catheter clamping may be tried. If the problem persists with significant residual volume, patient/attendants should be counselled and taught self or assisted clean intermittent catheterization. Also, cholinergic agents such as bethanechol (detrusor stimulation) or selective alpha 1 sympathetic clocker like tamsulosin (sphincter relaxation) may be tried and followed-up.[8,9]

Complications, Prevention, and Their Management

■ Neurological Injury

Approximately 3% of patients may have neurological worsening postsurgery, and it is more common in type I (Id) compared to type II. Injury usually occurs during removal of the bony spur, especially in disproportionate hemicords with oblique spurs overhanging them. This may be reduced by careful study of the preop imaging, identification of the morphology of the spur and adjacent anatomy, and accurate planning to avoid injury to the cord.

Also, wider laminectomy and piecemeal resections of the septum aid in reducing the injury and neurological deterioration.

■ CSF Leak and Pseudomeningocele

The most common and dreaded complication is CSF leak. There is no alternative to good dural closure technique. Spinal duramater should be preferably closed under microscope with a suture material no bigger than 4–0 in a continuous simple or continuous interlocking fashion.

Dural substitutes may be required in selected cases of lipoma where dura may be deficient and primary closure is not possible. Autologous grafts like thoracolumbar fascia, which can be obtained in the same incision, are preferred. Other agents like fascia lata, fat or muscle patch, and synthetic grafts may also be used.

Tissue glue may be used, but it only complements and does not replace good dural closure.

Once CSF leak has occurred, reinforcing sutures should be taken where necessary. A trial of pharmacological agents to reduce CSF production and reduce CSF pressure should be conducted– acetazolamide, spironolactone, and frusemide. If not controlled by these measures, the wound should be reexplored to identify the site of leak and close it.

Pseudomeningocele may be managed with pressure dressing. It need not be frequently tapped as it may introduce infection. It may be drained under aseptic precautions only if it is tense, and there is risk of rupture and CSF leak, and followed up with pressure dressing, prone nursing, acetazolamide, and frusemide.

■ Surgical Site Infections

Strict asepsis and thorough saline wash are key to avoiding surgical site infections.

■ Retethering

To prevent re-tethering we use fine monofilament (Prolene or ethilon 7 or 8–O) sutures for reconstructing the dura, as this decreases the raw area and prevents development of fibrotic bands. Moreover, it is also important to create an adequate sized dural sac to allow for free flow of CSF, which also offers protection from tethering.

References

1. Pang D, Dias MS, Ahab-Barmada M. Split cord malformation part I; Unified theory of embryogenesis for double spinal cord malformation. Neurosurgery 1992;31:451–460
2. Mahapatra AK, Gupta D. Split cord malformation: A clinical study of 254 patients and a proposal for a new clinical imaging classification. J Neurosurg 2006;103:531–536
3. Khandelwal A, Tandon V, Mahapatra AK. An unusual case of 4 level spinal dysraphism: multiple composite type 1 and type 2 split cord malformation, dorsal myelocystocele and hydrocephalous. J Pediatr Neurosci 2011;6(1):58–61

4. Erşahin Y, Mutluer S, Kocaman S, Demirtaş E. Split spinal cord malformations in children. J Neurosurg 1998;88(1):57–65

5. Borkar SA, Mahapatra AK. Split cord malformations: a two years experience at AIIMS. Asian J Neurosurg 2012;7(2):56–60

6. Sinha S, Agarwal D, Mahapatra AK. Split cord malformations: an experience of 203 cases. Childs Nerv Syst 2006;22(1):3–7

7. Akay KM, Izci Y, Baysefer A, Timurkaynak E. Split cord malformation in adults. Neurosurg Rev 2004;27(2):99–105

8. Geyik M, Geyik S, Şen H, et al. Urodynamic outcomes of detethering in children: experience with 46 pediatric patients. Childs Nerv Syst 2016;32(6):1079–1084

9. Kumar R, Singhal N, Gupta M, Kapoor R, Mahapatra AK. Evaluation of clinico-urodynamic outcome of bladder dysfunction after surgery in children with spinal dysraphism—a prospective study. Acta Neurochir (Wien) 2008;150(2):129–137

10. Erşahin Y. Split cord malformation types I and II: a personal series of 131 patients. Childs Nerv Syst 2013;29(9):1515–1526

11. Hoving EW, Haitsma E, Oude Ophuis CM, Journée HL. The value of intraoperative neurophysiological monitoring in tethered cord surgery. Childs Nerv Syst 2011;27(9):1445–1452

Long-Term Outcome of Split Cord Malformations

Manoj Phalak and Ashok K. Mahapatra

Table of Contents

■ Introduction 135

■ Axial Back Pain 135

■ Neurological Deficits 136

■ Orthopedic Deformity 136

■ Urological Symptoms 136

■ Causes of Postoperative Recurrence
  of Symptoms 136

■ Conclusion... 137

Long-Term Outcome of Split Cord Malformations

Manoj Phalak and Ashok K. Mahapatra

Introduction

Split cord malformation (SCM) is a type of neural tube defect in which the spinal cord is divided into two segments longitudinally. In 1992, Pang et al[1,2] proposed an embryogenic mechanism for this disorder and classified SCM into two types, which were earlier considered as two separate diseases.

Since then, there have been several classifications schemes for SCM.[3] The importance of these classification schemes comes from the fact that these may be related to the surgical plan as well as the immediate postoperative complications and long-term outcomes.

Surgery remains the mainstay of the treatment for all types of SCM amid some doubts regarding the need for surgery in asymptomatic type II SCM patients. However, with increasing age, the risk of developing neurological deficits increases in previously asymptomatic children.[4] Thus, surgery must be preferred for asymptomatic children as well. It must be ensured that surgery must not only take care of the fibrous and bony spur but also the associated pathologies like lipoma, teratoma, etc., which may be responsible for tethering.

In fact, on detailed evaluation, many such apparently asymptomatic children demonstrated signs of spinal cord dysfunction on objective testing like urodynamic studies. Unlike other etiologies of spinal cord tethering, there is paucity of literature regarding the long-term outcomes of SCM after surgical correction.

If all the tethering elements are surgically released and associated pathologies are taken care of, the outcomes of surgery for SCM are generally considered to be good. However, Pang et al[5] observed significant incidence of associated ventral tethering, which must be removed to avoid the need for repeat surgery. MRI is not a sensitive investigation for detecting ventral tethering, and CT myelography is considered to be a better method for the same.[5]

The long-term outcomes of SCM can be discussed in terms of progression of the symptoms of spinal cord dysfunction and the need for repeat surgery due to retethering or reformation of spur, resulting in the recurrence of the symptoms or deterioration in previously stable neurological deficit.

In most of the studies, improvement or stabilization of symptoms has been reported in >90% of patients.[2,3,6,7]

Axial Back Pain

Axial back pain improves or stabilizes in the majority of the patients.[1,8] This improvement may sometimes be confounded by factors like complexity of SCM, which is associated with greater incidence of retethering and progressive orthopedic deformity after surgery.[6]

Neurological Deficits

More than 90% of those who present with neurological deficits preoperatively either experience complete or partial resolution of symptoms or the symptoms remain stable.[6] In the remaining 10% of patients, there is risk of further deterioration. However, no patient who was initially asymptomatic has been reported to suffer neurological deterioration after an uneventful surgery.[3] This observation along with the natural progression of disease lends strength to the consensus opinion favoring operative intervention in even the asymptomatic patients.

Orthopedic Deformity

Most of the cases with significant scoliosis and spinal deformity end up requiring a spinal stabilization procedure early in their lives.[9] The surgery done for SCM and detethering has no role in halting the progression of orthopedic deformity. Hence, the risk of development of neurological symptoms as a part of neuro-orthopedic syndrome is not affected by detethering alone.[10] This is in consensus with the observations regarding associated orthopedic deformities in other etiologies of tethered cord like myelomeningocele.[9]

Urological Symptoms

Urological symptoms are expected to improve in at least a third of the patients after surgery.[11] However, it is very common for subtle urological abnormalities to be missed in the preoperative evaluation unless routine preoperative urodynamic studies are done. Patients with such a degree of urological symptoms usually report stabilization or improvement of symptoms.[12]

It is recommended that urodynamic studies must be done in all the patients.[13] Other than being an objective parameter to assess the impact of surgery, it is a sensitive indicator for retethering, which may present with reappearance of urological symptoms or asymptomatic abnormalities in urodynamic testing.

Causes of Postoperative Recurrence of Symptoms

■ Missed Secondary Tethering Lesion (Complex SCM)

According to Pang et al,[1] SCM is almost always associated with a secondary tethering lesion. In the literature, the rate of secondary tethering lesions associated with SCM varies from 50 to 100%.[14,15] Considering such high rates of these lesions, it is imperative that the patients' radiography findings are thoroughly evaluated for presence of such lesions. Proctor et al[6] found secondary lesions to be associated in 69% of their patients, with fatty filum being the most common, followed by lipoma. It is also observed that at the site of split, the cord may have arachnoid bands extending dorsally and cephalad, tethering it.[3] These associated tethering lesions must be taken care of in the initial surgery. Otherwise, there is high likelihood of recurrence or worsening of symptoms as a result of tethering of the cord.

■ Retethering

The rate of retethering after surgery for SCM is around 10% in various reports. Mahapatra et al[3] report a retethering rate of 7 to 10% over a follow-up period of 5 years in their study of 300 patients. Similarly, Proctor et al[6] report retethering in two out of 16 patients (12.5%). This retethering may be due to regrowth of spur, postoperative arachnoiditis, or a secondary tethering lesion left unattended in the first surgery.[3,6,16] For early detection of retethering, it is advisable to do routine interval postoperative urodynamic testing, which detects bladder dysfunction prior to appearance of urological symptoms.[13] Radiographic appearance of retethering must always be interpreted with clinical sign and symptoms. In patients with symptoms of tethering on clinical grounds, MRI may help in locating the tethering element. Enlarging syringomyelia is also an indirect indicator of retethering and portends risk of clinical worsening.[8]

■ Regrowth of Spur

Gupta et al[16] in 2010 reported a case in which there was regrowth of the bony spur. They observed that the dural sleeve, which was not excised during the initial surgery, provided scaffolding for probably the mesenchymal elements that led to reformation of the bony spur at the same site. Although the patient initially improved after surgery but presented 9 years later with progressive lower limb weakness due to regrowth of spur. Thus, regrowth of spur may be one of the causes of retethering, leading to delayed neurological progression after surgery.

Conclusion

Long-term outcomes of SCM after surgery generally seem favorable. However, there is high rate of recurrence or progression of symptoms if associated causes of tethering are overlooked in the first surgery. There is significant reduction or stabilization of all the symptoms including axial back pain, neurological deficits, and bladder symptoms. However, surgery has no role in preventing the progression of orthopedic deformity and a significant number of patients require scoliosis correction later in life.

References

1. Pang D. Split cord malformation: Part II: Clinical syndrome. Neurosurgery 1992;31(3):481–500
2. Pang D, Dias MS, Ahab-Barmada M. Split cord malformation: Part I: A unified theory of embryogenesis for double spinal cord malformations. Neurosurgery 1992;31(3):451–480
3. Mahapatra AK. Split cord malformation—A study of 300 cases at AIIMS 1990–2006. J Pediatr Neurosci 2011;6(Suppl 1):S41–S45
4. Yamada S, Zinke DE, Sanders D. Pathophysiology of "tethered cord syndrome." J Neurosurg 1981;54(4):494–503
5. Pang D. Ventral tethering in split cord malformation. Neurosurg Focus 2001;10(1):e6
6. Proctor MR, Scott RM. Long-term outcome for patients with split cord malformation. Neurosurg Focus 2001;10(1):e5
7. Raskin JS, Litvack ZN, Selden NR. Split spinal cord. In: Winn HR, Youmans JR, eds. Youmans and Winn Neurological Surgery. 7th ed. Philadelphia, PA: Elsevier; 2017:1842–1848

8. Kaminker R, Fabry J, Midha R, Finkelstein JA. Split cord malformation with diastematomyelia presenting as neurogenic claudication in an adult: a case report. Spine 2000;25(17):2269–2271

9. Pierz K, Banta J, Thomson J, Gahm N, Hartford J. The effect of tethered cord release on scoliosis in myelomeningocele. J Pediatr Orthop 2000;20(3):362–365

10. Andar UB, Harkness WFJ, Hayward RD. Split cord malformations of the lumbar region. A model for the neurosurgical management of all types of "occult" spinal dysraphism? Pediatr Neurosurg 1997;26(1):17–24

11. Mahapatra AK, Gupta DK. Split cord malformations: a clinical study of 254 patients and a proposal for a new clinical-imaging classification. J Neurosurg 2005; 103(6, Suppl):531–536

12. Proctor MR, Bauer SB, Scott RM. The effect of surgery for split spinal cord malformation on neurologic and urologic function. Pediatr Neurosurg 2000;32(1):13–19

13. Pérez LM, Barnes N, MacDiarmid SA, Oakes WJ, Webster GD. Urological dysfunction in patients with diastematomyelia. J Urol 1993;149(6):1503–1505

14. Ersahin Y, Mutluer S, Kocaman S, Demirtas E. Split spinal cord malformations in children. Neurosurg Focus 1997;3:E1

15. Jindal A, Mahapatra AK. Split cord malformations—a clinical study of 48 cases. Indian Pediatr 2000;37(6):603–607

16. Gupta DK, Ahmed S, Garg K, Mahapatra AK. Regrowth of septal spur in split cord malformation. Pediatr Neurosurg 2010;46(3):242–244

Anesthesia for Neural Tube Defects

Ashutosh Kaushal and Ashish Bindra

Table of Contents

- Introduction 141
- Preanesthetic Evaluation 141
- Systemic Evaluation 141
- Airway and Respiratory Evaluation 142
- Perioperative Investigations 142
- Preanesthetic Preparation 143
- OT Preparation 144
- Induction of General Anesthesia 144
- Anesthesia Technique... 145
- Intraoperative Fluid Management 146
- Intraoperative Blood Transfusion 147
- Intraoperative Systemic Complications 147
- Postoperative Care 148
- Conclusions 148

Anesthesia for Neural Tube Defects

Ashutosh Kaushal and Ashish Bindra

Introduction

Neural tube defects (NTDs) are a consequence of nonfusion of neural tube during the first few weeks of intrauterine development. The defects may range from relatively benign conditions to abnormalities involving vertebral bodies, spinal cord, and brainstem incompatible with life. Meningocele (herniation of the meninges), meningomyelocele (MMC; herniation of the elements of the neural tube), encephaloceles, and spina bifida are open NTDs whereas lipomyelomeningocele, lipomeningocele, and SCM are common examples of closed NTDs. Early surgical repair is warranted to minimize risk of infection, development of hydrocephalus, cerebrospinal fluid (CSF) leakage, and further neurological damage. NTDs may be associated with other congenital anomalies. Many such patients present in the early neonatal period for primary closure of defect, making the procedure challenging for both the surgeon and the anesthesiologist.

This chapter discusses the anesthetic and perioperative concerns of pediatric patients presenting for repair of all NTDs and not restricted to SCM alone. Besides inherent risks of anesthesia and surgery in the pediatric population, special considerations pertaining to disease, non-neurological complications, and perioperative management of associated systemic anomalies will be discussed in this chapter.

Preanesthetic Evaluation

To minimize infection of the exposed cord and consequent sepsis, open NTDS are repaired as early as possible within the first few days of life.[1] The preoperative visit is the first interaction of an anesthesiologist with a patient. A neonate should be evaluated for all possible anomalies during this visit. It is the only time for an anesthesiologist to build a rapport with older children, especially toddlers. For planning good anesthesia technique, a thorough history and physical examination to look for neurological and systemic abnormalities is a must. A proper history and examination can rule out involvement of other systems. In the presence of specific symptoms, required investigations should be requested and documented. Patient physiology should be optimized to as normal as possible without undue delay in surgical procedure.

Systemic Evaluation

NTDs are frequently associated with other anomalies, including heart, esophagus, kidneys, brain, limbs, and anal canal. Congenital heart disease (atrial and ventricular septal defects, anomalous pulmonary venous circulation, dextrocardia, patent ductus arteriosus, tetralogy of Fallot, bicuspid aortic valve, coarctation, and hypoplastic left heart syndrome) may be present in up to 37% patients with NTDs.[2] History of recurrent chest infections, cyanotic spells, and abnormal auscultation of heart along with

X-ray findings suggestive of cardiac involvement mandate cardiac evaluation by an expert. Preoperative echocardiography is advised to assess cardiac function in these patients. Anorectal malformations, hydronephrosis, tracheoesophageal fistula, hydroureter, malformed ureters, solitary kidney, horseshoe kidney, neurogenic bladder, exstrophy of bladder, undescended testes, hydrocele, omphalocele, Meckel's diverticulum, and inguinal hernia are the other common problems seen in these children. Genitourinary anomalies are seen in up to 10 to 30% of the patients.[3] Presence of facial cleft, kyphoscoliosis, and chest wall malformation may pose problems during intubation, positioning, and ventilation of these patients and make perioperative period challenging. Other neurological anomalies like Arnold–Chiari II malformation, hydrocephalus, microcephaly, corpus callosum agenesis, Dandy–Walker malformation, Meckel syndrome, microgyria, porencephalic cyst, arachnoid cyst, and vitreous degeneration commonly accompany NTDs. Infants with hydrocephalus and Arnold–Chiari malformation are prone to cervical cord compression during extension of spine and may develop severe bradycardia at the time of laryngoscopy and intubation. According to a retrospective analysis of 135 children with MMC, hydrocephalus was the most common association (67.4%), followed by Chiari-II malformation (58.4%). Renal abnormality was present in 9% of cases and 24.4% of children had scoliosis. Two infants (1.5%) presented with inspiratory stridor. Two children (1.5%) suffered cardiac arrest; both had associated Chiari-II malformation and hydrocephalus. Postoperative ventilation was required in 8.9% of children, primarily due to inadequate reversal from neuromuscular blockade.[4]

Raised intracranial pressure (ICP) and preoperative drowsiness may contribute to delayed awakening after surgery. Lower cranial nerve palsies may result in aspiration pneumonia and prolonged ventilatory requirement. Serum electrolytes abnormalities, especially sodium and potassium, are commonly seen in patients with frequent vomiting episodes. If CSF shunt is present, its function should always be assessed before induction of anesthesia. Choice of anesthetic agent and perioperative course can be anticipated and properly planned with complete knowledge of patient profile.

Airway and Respiratory Evaluation

Securing airway is difficult in neonates and infants when compared to adults. It becomes even more difficult in the presence of midline swelling, large hydrocephalic head and facial clefts. Ventilation can be rendered difficult due to big nasal encephalocele. Patients with Arnold–Chiari have irregular control of ventilation, impaired chemical drive, and bilateral vocal cord paralysis. Such patients may present with apneic spells. Patients can suffer from aspiration pneumonia attributable to gastroesophageal reflux, absent gag and cough reflexes, or lack of oropharyngeal coordination.[5] Short trachea is present in 36% of patients with MMC.[6] Postoperative mechanical ventilation should be anticipated in patients with abdominal muscle weakness and inefficient cough, causing decreased ability to clear secretions after prolonged surgery.[5] It should be discussed with guardians. Infants which are irritable, lethargic, and with altered consciousness may remain so postoperatively, and extubation plan may be decided accordingly.

Perioperative Investigations

Routine and specific investigations depending on the systems involved should be obtained. Baseline hemogram and leukocyte count are done if not done in the previous 1 month. Raised leucocyte count indicates an infected sac. Blood grouping and cross-matching are advisable in case of large defect, warranting perioperative blood transfusion. Adequate amount of blood and blood product should be arranged.

Chest X-ray is useful to rule out cardiomegaly in suspicious cases. It may also help to identify any evidence of aspiration. Air bronchogram is considered to see the length of trachea.[6] Electrocardiography (ECG) and 2D echocardiography may help to delineate underlying cardiac anomalies. Additional studies should include coagulation profile and renal and hepatic function as per requirement.

Preanesthetic Preparation

Fasting instructions: When determining a suitable fasting period, both the amount and nature of foods ingested must be considered. Preoperative fasting guidelines recommended by American Society of Anesthesiologists (ASA) task force are shown in **Table 14.1**. For elective surgeries, pediatric patients should preferably be kept first in the list.[7]

Premedication: The requirement of type of premedication depends on the neurological status and the age of patient. Baby may be shifted carefully to or in the lap of a nurse. The swelling should be handled with gloved hands and cotton pads. Toddler paranesthesia room can be equipped with toys and popular animation movies. Anxiolysis is seldom required for neonates; however, anxiolytics are essential in an infant to allay separation anxiety. Benzodiazepines are the preferred drugs. Oversedation may result in hypoventilation and augmentation of ICP, causing brainstem herniation, especially in patients with Arnold–Chiari malformation, so medication should be administered under strict supervision only.

■ Latex Sensitivity

The reported incidence of latex allergy and latex sensitization in patients with MMC is 10 to 73%.[8–10] The potential reasons include contact to latex products during repeated bladder catheterizations, genetic propensity, and multiple surgical procedures. The manifestation of allergic reactions can be mild (tingling of the lips, facial swelling, and wheezing) to severe anaphylaxis with cardiovascular collapse. Children with a possibility for latex sensitivity and anaphylaxis should be managed in latex-free setting, and if anaphylaxis develop during surgery, latex allergy should be suspected. Removal of the latex, administration of fluid, and treatment for anaphylaxis like intravenous epinephrine, vasopressors, steroids, H1 and H2 histamine blockers should be administered, depending upon the symptomatology.[11]

Table 14.1 Fasting guidelines for pediatric patients

Ingested material	Minimum fasting period
Clear liquids	2 h
Breast milk	4 h
Infant formula	6 h
Nonhuman milk	6 h
Light meal	6 h
Fried foods, fatty foods, or meat	≥ 8h

OT Preparation

Hypothermia prevention: Thin skin, low fat content, exposure of large body surface area, cold irrigation fluid, skin preparation, prolonged wound exposure, general anesthesia (GA)-induced redistribution of heat from core to periphery, administration of intravenous (IV) fluid at room temperature, irrigation fluid, and dry anesthetic gases are major factors responsible for development of intraoperative hypothermia in the pediatric population. Premature patients with large lesions have inherent difficulty in maintaining body temperature. Hypothermia may cause delayed awakening from anesthesia, cardiac irritability, respiratory depression, increased pulmonary vascular resistance, and altered responses to intraoperative anesthetics and neuromuscular blocking agents.

The risk of hypothermia can be decreased by warming operating theatre ≥26° before shifting the patient to operating room. Using heated humidified inspired gases and warming all IV and irrigation fluids helps to minimize the heat loss. The patient's limbs and uninvolved body area should be covered to maintain body temperature.[12] Passive warming devices (cotton blankets, surgical drapes, plastic sheets, reflective composites, sleeping bags) or active warming devices (circulating water mattresses/garments, force air warmers, resistive heating devices, negative pressure water warming systems, and radiant heaters) can be used to keep the child warm.

Induction of General Anesthesia

Preparation of weight-calculated drugs, airway cart, pediatric breathing circuit, etc., should be ensured before arrival of the patient.

Proper positioning during induction of GA and surgery is of utmost importance, as neonates with hydrocephalus show a diminished response to hypoxia and increased susceptibility to postoperative apnea.[13] Any direct pressure on the uncovered neural placode adds to neural insult.[14] Infants with hydrocephalus and Arnold–Chiari malformation are more prone to cervical cord compression during extension for intubation. Positioning and airway management are specially challenging in case of large encephalocele. For induction, patient can be placed in supine or lateral position, depending on size and site of the defect. Foam cushion devices are also described for protecting the fragile sac from being compressed.[15] Additional padding beneath the shoulders and head may be needed if placing the defect in the middle of a "doughnut" causes pressure on the open defect.[16] Babies with large head can have their head dangling (well-supported by an assistant) over the edge of table for intubation purpose. Head dangling avoids pressure on the encephalocele sac[17] and attains proper positioning for intubation. Head can be placed over horseshoe head holder to avoid direct compression of the defect (**Fig. 14.1**). Chance of compression of the sac, and hence a raised ICP, can also be avoided by intubation in lateral position.[18]

Difficult airway should be anticipated in syndromic babies with abnormal facies. Preoxygenation with a nonlatex mask of appropriate size is advised. In patients with facial deformity, prevention of sac compression during mask ventilation is essential. Modification of mask ventilation can be used for it.[19]

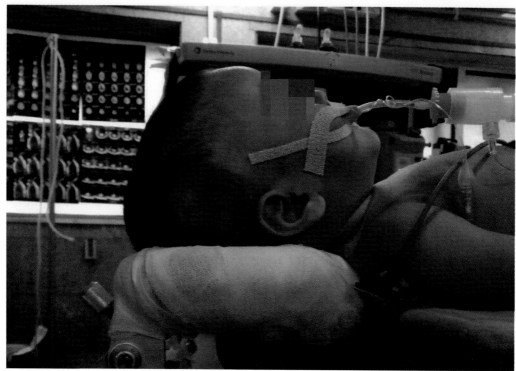

Fig. 14.1 Patient head positioned over horseshoe.

Anesthesia Technique

The goal of anesthetic induction is to avoid hypoxia, hypercapnia, and volatile anesthetic-induced increases in cerebral blood flow, as all these factors may increase ICP. Other considerations are related to difficult positioning and associated anomalies and congenital malformations. The trachea may be intubated after the IV administration of a sedative-hypnotic and an intermediate acting nondepolarizing muscle relaxant. An IV induction with thiopentone or propofol is commonly practiced. However, in children without IV access or with difficult IV access, inhalational induction by facemask with sevoflurane is preferred to avoid crying and struggling.[20] IV technique may be continued after IV access is secured. Succinylcholine should be avoided in patients with neurological deficit. The indication of awake intubation is unusual positioning and anticipated very difficult airway. An international consensus group and others have raised concerns about awake intubation until it is a life-threatening condition.[16] At the time of laryngoscopy and induction, children may develop bradycardia due to brainstem compression. Since short trachea has been described in children with MMC, it is essential to prevent endobronchial migration of tracheal tubes. After induction, the patient is made prone on an adequate-sized bolster, head is well-supported, and all bony points and eyes are padded. Abdomen should be free of any external compression (**Fig. 14.2**).

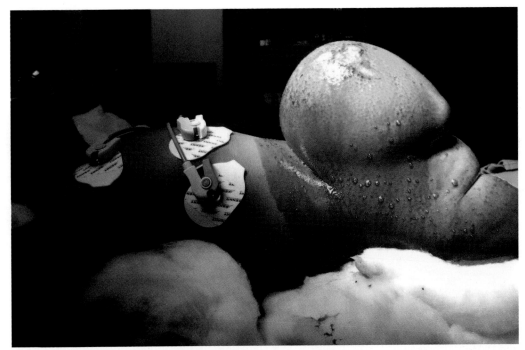

Fig. 14.2 Patient under anesthesia in prone position.

The choice of anesthetic agents is decided by the type of surgery and the intraoperative neuro-monitoring (IONM) modality used, because all anesthetic agents affect synaptic function. Halogenated volatile agents should be avoided in modalities that involve cortical tracts, since they decrease evoked potential amplitude and increase latency. The most commonly used technique is total IV anesthesia that is a combination of propofol with opioids (fentanyl/remifentanil). Although muscle relaxants do not affect somatosensory-evoked potentials (SSEPs), they inhibit motor-evoked potentials (MEPs); hence, they should be avoided during multimodal monitoring. Significant increases in ICP or reductions in hematocrit, blood volume, carbon dioxide, and oxygenation and hypothermia are physiological variables that may alter responses during IONM and should be kept stable and within normal limits.[21,22] Low concentration of inhalational agent (minimum alveolar concentration [MAC] <1) and a narcotic appropriate to the length of the procedure can also be used to maintain anesthesia. Muscle relaxant is particularly avoided in cases planned for IONM.

Intraoperative Fluid Management

The intraoperative goal is to maintain normovolemia and hemodynamic stability. An infusion pump or a burette with a microdrip chamber should be used for accurate measurements of fluid, because pediatric patients have limited margins for error. According to present recommendations, balanced isotonic salt solution should be used for fasting deficit, intraoperative background infusion, and third space losses.

Maintenance requirements per hour for pediatric patients can be calculated by Holliday and Segar "4:2:1" rule.[23] Hypotonic maintenance fluids like 5% dextrose should be avoided, as they may cause hyponatremia, cerebral edema, and encephalopathy. Intraoperative fluids meant for background infusion should have osmolarity, sodium and metabolic anions near to physiological range. One to 2.5% glucose may be added to the maintenance fluid.[24] These kinds of solution avoid both hypo and hyperglycemia and prevent lipolysis.[25] The replacement of fasting deficit is no longer important as per new fasting guidelines. Now, it is evident that despite prolonged fasting, healthy patients can maintain normal volumes and blood sugar.[26,27] In recent years, there has been increasing data suggestive of poorer outcomes with excessive use of intraoperative fluid. Blood loss should be simultaneously replaced by either colloid or packed red cells.[28] Fluid inside the encephalocele sac comprises third space fluid shift and not in direct continuation with the systemic circulation; thus, it does not need replacement. Dyselectrolytemia due to aspiration of large volumes of CSF, hypothermia, and blood loss may develop and should be managed appropriately.

Intraoperative Blood Transfusion

Estimation of blood loss in pediatric patients is difficult. Amount of blood in the suction container and visual assessment of the blood on surgical sponges and lap sponges are commonly used for estimation of blood loss. A completely wet standard size surgical sponge and lap sponge hold approximately 10 mL and 100 to 150 mL of blood, respectively. Hemoglobin concentrations in serial arterial blood gases (ABG) imitate the ratio of blood cells to plasma and not essentially reflect the actual amount of blood lost. Potential or actual ongoing rate and magnitude of bleeding, intravascular volume status, signs of organ ischemia, and adequacy of cardiopulmonary reserve are the major factors determining red blood cell transfusion. Generally, transfusion should begin after 10 to 20% blood volume loss in a patient with a normal preoperative hematocrit. The exact trigger point depends on the patient's medical state and the surgical procedure. Transfusion should be considered when blood loss exceeds minimal allowable blood loss (MABL).

MABL = 3 × estimated blood volume × (preoperative hematocrit − transfusion trigger hematocrit).

Blood transfusion is recommended at hematocrit of ≤24%. However, it is also important to take into account the rate of blood loss and comorbid conditions. Red blood cells transfusion (10 mL/kg) increases the hematocrit by approximately 10% in neonates.[28] Early blood transfusion is indicated in phase of massive ongoing blood loss.

Intraoperative Systemic Complications

Various intraoperative complications reported include hemodynamic disturbances in the form of bradycardia, tachycardia, hypotension, and arrhythmias. Pediatric patients are prone to hypoxemia, hypercarbia, bronchospasm, and tracheal tube displacement, especially during prone position. Cardiac arrest due to sudden loss of CSF from sac, causing traction of cerebral neuronal pathways involving brainstem nuclei, has been reported.[29-31]

■ Reversal

The goal is "rapid awakening" in order to help early neurological assessment, hemodynamic stability, and minimize coughing and straining. Adequate reversal of neuromuscular blockade should be attained before extubating the patient. The neonate's trachea may be extubated after short and uncomplicated procedures when the patient is fully awake and breathing well at the end of the procedure, and neurologic integrity has been confirmed. Hypothermia is a common cause of delayed awakening in pediatric patients. Other anesthetic causes include inadequate reversal, residual effect of anesthetic agents, and dyselectrolytemia. Neurosurgical complications should also be ruled out in such cases.

Postoperative Care

All infants, especially preterm infants < 50 weeks postconceptual age and patients with obstructive sleep apnea, are at risk of postoperative hypoventilation and apnea and should be monitored with plethysmograph and apnea monitors in intensive care units. Respiratory difficulties may occur after a tight primary closure, following repair of a large skin defect.[32] The ventilatory response to hypoxia and hypercarbia may be weak or absent particularly in patients with hydrocephalus and Chiari malformation. Postoperative chest radiograph to confirm the correct position of the endotracheal tube should be done to avoid accidental endobronchial intubation and subsequent problems in patients with tracheal tube in situ. Brainstem dysfunction due to associated Arnold–Chiari malformation may cause stridor, dysphagia, cranial nerve dysfunction, and central hypoventilation.[33] Structural changes in different pathways of respiratory control leads to hypoventilation, sleep apnea, and prolonged breath holding.[5,34] Bilateral vocal cord paralysis may complicate respiratory recovery. Reasons for postoperative mechanical ventilation include inadequate recovery, hypothermia or respiratory issues. In a study of 118 children who underwent excision and repair of encephalocele over a period of 10 years, only 16 required postoperative ventilation.[31]

Patients should be nursed in a lateral position. Hypothermia should be prevented. Infiltration of the wound at the end of surgery with local anesthetic provides pain relief in the immediate postoperative period. Paracetamol is a commonly used analgesic in the form of IV formulation or rectal suppository. Opioids can be supplemented if there are no contraindications to their use and good nursing care is available.

Conclusions

Patients presenting to or for repair of NTDs may range from neonate to adolescent. Age-related physiology and disease-related pathophysiology should be kept in mind while delivering anesthesia to them (**Table 14.2**). Carefully planned anesthetic technique decreases perioperative morbidity and mortality.

Table 14.2 Anesthetic concerns in patients with NTDs

Stage of evaluation	Related concerns
Preoperative evaluation	• Complete workup to rule out associated anomalies • Evaluation and documentation of neurological deficits • Size and location of defect and its effect on anesthesia and positioning • Complete airway and respiratory assessment • Cardiovascular assessment • Evaluation for need of postoperative ventilation • History of latex sensitivity • Appropriate preoperative investigations
Intraoperative concerns	**Proper positioning** • To avoid direct pressure on defect • Avoid excessive extension during intubation • Check tracheal tube position, and prevent kinking and endobronchial migration • Ensure patient safety in prone position **Anesthetic technique to ensure** • Adequate depth of anesthesia • Hemodynamic stability • Intraoperative neuromonitoring • Rapid wakening at the end of procedure **Avoid** • Hypothermia • Hypovolemia • Hyponatremia • Hypercarbia
Postoperative considerations	• Intensive nursing care • Analgesia • Hypothermia prevention

Abbreviation: NTDs, neural tube defects.

References

1. Soundararajan N, Cunliffe M. Anaesthesia for spinal surgery in children. Br J Anaesth 2007;99(1): 86–94
2. Koçak G, Onal C, Koçak A, et al. Prevalence and outcome of congenital heart disease in patients with neural tube defect. J Child Neurol 2008;23(5):526–530
3. Pérez LM, Wilbanks JT, Joseph DB, Oakes WJ. Urological outcome of patients with cervical and upper thoracic myelomeningocele. J Urol 2000;164:962–964
4. Singh D, Rath GP, Dash HH, Bithal PK. Anesthetic concerns and perioperative complications in repair of myelomeningocele: a retrospective review of 135 cases. J Neurosurg Anesthesiol 2010;22(1): 11–15
5. Oren J, Kelly DH, Todres ID, Shannon DC. Respiratory complications in patients with myelodysplasia and Arnold-Chiari malformation. Am J Dis Child 1986;140(3):221–224
6. Wells TR, Jacobs RA, Senac MO, Landing BH. Incidence of short trachea in patients with myelomeningocele. Pediatr Neurol 1990;6(2):109–111

7. ASA Task Force on preoperative fasting. Practice Guidelines for Preoperative Fasting and the Use of Pharmacologic Agents to Reduce the Risk of Pulmonary Aspiration. Application to Healthy Patients Undergoing Elective Procedures Anesthesiology 2017;126:376–393

8. Chen Z, Cremer R, Baur X. Latex allergy correlates with operation. Allergy 1997;52(8):873

9. Kelly KJ, Pearson ML, Kurup VP, et al. A cluster of anaphylactic reactions in children with spina bifida during general anesthesia: epidemiologic features, risk factors, and latex hypersensitivity. J Allergy Clin Immunol 1994;94(1):53–61

10. Ellsworth P, Merguerian P, Klein R, et al. Evaluation and risk factors of latex allergy in spina bifida patients: is it preventable? J Urol 1993;150:691–693

11. Newfield P, Cottrell JE. Handbook of Neuroanaesthsia. 5th ed. Philadelphia, PA: Lippincott Williams & Wilkins; 2012:273

12. Bindu B, Bindra A, Rath G. Temperature management under general anesthesia: compulsion or option. J Anaesthesiol Clin Pharmacol 2017;33(3):306–316

13. Bell WO, Charney EB, Bruce DA, Sutton LN, Schut L. Symptomatic Arnold-Chiari malformation: review of experience with 22 cases. J Neurosurg 1987;66(6):812–816

14. McLone DG, Knepper PA. The cause of Chiari II malformation: a unified theory. Pediatr Neurosci 1989;15(1):1–12

15. Quezado Z, Finkel JC. Airway management in neonates with occipital encephalocele: easy does it. Anesth Analg 2008;107(4):1446

16. Horiki T. Anesthesia during surgery for meningomyelocele. Neuroanesthesia and cerebrospinal protection. Tokyo: Springer; 2015:543–549

17. Dey N, Gombar KK, Khanna AK, Khandelwal P. Airway management in neonates with occipital encephalocele: adjustments and modifications. Paediatr Anaesth 2007;17(11):1119–1120

18. Creighton RE, Relton JES, Meridy HW. Anaesthesia for occipital encephalocoele. Can Anaesth Soc J 1974;21(4):403–406

19. Mahajan C, Rath GP. Anaesthetic management in a child with frontonasal encephalocele. J Anaesthesiol Clin Pharmacol 2010;26(4):570–571

20. Furay C, Howell T. Paediatric neuroanaesthesia. Contin Educ Anaesth Crit Care Pain 2010;10: 172–176

21. Rath GP, Dash HH. Anaesthesia for neurosurgical procedures in paediatric patients. Indian J Anaesth 2012;56(5):502–510

22. Sloan T. Anesthesia and intraoperative neurophysiological monitoring in children. Childs Nerv Syst 2010;26(2):227–235

23. Holliday MA, Segar WE. The maintenance need for water in parenteral fluid therapy. Pediatrics 1957;19(5):823–832

24. Sümpelmann R, Becke K, Crean P, et al. German Scientific Working Group for Paediatric Anaesthesia. European consensus statement for intraoperative fluid therapy in children. Eur J Anaesthesiol 2011;28(9):637–639

25. Sümpelmann R, Becke K, Brenner S, et al. Perioperative intravenous fluid therapy in children: guidelines from the Association of the Scientific Medical Societies in Germany. Paediatr Anaesth 2017;27(1):10–18

26. Jacob M, Chappell D, Conzen P, Finsterer U, Rehm M. Blood volume is normal after pre-operative overnight fasting. Acta Anaesthesiol Scand 2008;52(4):522–529

27. Bailey AG, McNaull PP, Jooste E, Tuchman JB. Perioperative crystalloid and colloid fluid management in children: Where are we and how did we get here. Anesth Analg 2010;110(2):375–390

28. Mackey DC, Butterworth JF, Mikhail MS, Morgan GE, Wasnick JD. Morgan & Mikhail's Clinical Anesthesiology. 5th ed. New York, NY: McGraw-Hill Education LLC; 2013

29. Ganjoo P, Kaushik S. An unexpected complication of encephalocele repair. J Neurosurg Anesthesiol 1993;5(2):137–138

30. Rickert CH, Grabellus F, Varchmin-Schultheiss K, Stöss H, Paulus W. Sudden unexpected death in young adults with chronic hydrocephalus. Int J Legal Med 2001;114(6):331–337
31. Mahajan C, Rath GP, Dash HH, Bithal PK. Perioperative management of children with encephalocele: an institutional experience. J Neurosurg Anesthesiol 2011;23(4):352–356
32. Chouhan RS, Bindra A, Mishra N, Hasija N, Sinha S. A rare case of abdominal compartment syndrome following repair of large myelomeningocele. J Pediatr Neurosci 2015;10(4):365–367
33. Ward SL, Jacobs RA, Gates EP, Hart LD, Keens TG. Abnormal ventilatory patterns during sleep in infants with myelomeningocele. J Pediatr 1986;109(4):631–634
34. Petersen MC, Wolraich M, Sherbondy A, Wagener J. Abnormalities in control of ventilation in newborn infants with myelomeningocele. J Pediatr 1995;126(6):1011–1015

Index

A

Accessory neurenteric canal, 12, 24
Active warming devices, 144
Adult split cord malformation
    clinical features
        backache, 95, 95f
        hypertrichosis, 96
        level of split, 96
        orthopedic abnormalities, 96
        sensorimotor deficits, 95
    demography, 91–94
    imaging, 96
    literature on management and outcomes
        reported in, 92–94t
    pathophysiology, 91
    treatment and outcome, 96–97
Airway and respiratory evaluation, 142
Anesthetic agents, choice of, 146
Anesthetic concerns, in patients with NTDs, 149t
    airway and respiratory evaluation, 142
    choice of anesthetic agents, 146
    fasting guidelines for pediatric patients, 143t
    induction of general anesthesia, 144–145
    intraoperative blood transfusion, 147
    intraoperative fluid management, 145–146
    intraoperative systemic complications, 147–148
    latex sensitivity, 143
    OT preparation, 144
    perioperative investigations, 142–143
    postoperative care, 148
    preanesthetic evaluation, 141
    preanesthetic preparation, 143
    in prone position, 146f
    reversal, 148
    systemic evaluation, 141–142
Anorectal malformation, 104
Axial back pain, 135

B

Bony spur, hypotheses for posterior origin of, 12

C

Cervical split cord malformations
    antenatal diagnosis, 72
    clinical symptoms, 72
    documented cases of, 66–71t
    embryology, 63–64
    epidemiology, 64–65
    familial inheritance pattern, 65
    pathophysiology of symptoms, 64
    postnatal diagnosis, 72–73
    surgical management
        complications, 74–75

indications for, 73
    IONM, 73
    laminoplasty, 74
    laminotomy, 73–74
    outcome, 74
    pedicle screw fixation, 74
    urodynamic evaluation, 73
Complex SCM
    classification of, 101
    clinical presentation, 104
    embryogenesis, 102–104
    encountered in clinical practice, 101–102
    with intraspinal teratoma, 103
    investigations, 104–105
    treatment, 105–106
Complex spina bifida, 101
Complex spinal dysraphism, 81, 101
    associated with anomalies of organ systems,
        104
    clinical spectrum covered under, 101
    multicomponent, 103–104
    multilevel, 104
Composite SCM, 19–20, 20f, 103
    cases of, 83–84
    clinical findings, 84
    clinical significance, 83
    complex spinal dysraphic abnormality in, 81
    distribution of spurs in, 83
    embryogenesis, 82
    incidence of, 82, 103
    occurrence of, 102
    single stage surgery for, 84–85
Congenital scoliosis, 25
Cranial dysraphisms
    congenital malformations, 21
    open form of, 21
    SCMs associated with, 21–22
CSF leak, 129
CT scan, 123
Cutaneous markers, 54

D

Detethering operation, 115
Diastematomyelia, 31, 53, 63
Diplomyelia, 17, 53, 63
Dorsal spur
    clinical features, 54
    demography, 54
    embryology, 53–54
    with HPA, 54
    imaging studies, 57
    literature review of SCM cases with, 55t, 56t
    mechanisms for occurrence of, 64

patient outcome, 58
treatment, 57–58

E
Embryogenesis of SCM, 3–4, 24–25, 53
    gastrulation, 9–10
    notochord formation, 10–12
    SCM type I, 12
    unified theory on, 12, 53–54
Endomesenchymal tract, 3–4, 12, 43
Epiblast cells, 9–10
Extracranial malformations, spur with, 23

F
Fasting guidelines for pediatric patients, 143*t*
Filum terminale transection, 129

G
Gastrulation, midline axial integration during, 12
General anesthesia, induction of, 144–145

H
Hemimyelomeningocele, 103
Human embryo development
    gastrulation, 9–10
    notochord formation, 10–12
        fusion with endoderm, 10
        neural tube formation, 10–11
        neurenteric canal formation, 10, 11*f*
        secondary neurulation, 11–12
        spinal neurocele occlusion, 12
Hydrocephalus (HCP), child with, 22*f*
Hypothermia prevention, 144

I
Intracranial malformations, spur with, 23
Intradural pathologies, 128
Intraoperative blood transfusion, 147
Intraoperative fluid management, 145–146
Intraoperative neurophysiological monitoring
    (IONM)
    for adult SCM, 96
    for cervical SCM, 73
Intraoperative systemic complications, 147–148

L
Laminectomy
    and isolation of spur, 126–127
    and laminotomy, 128
Laminoplasty, 74
Laminotomy, for cervical SCM, 73–74
Latex sensitivity, 143
Long-term outcomes of SCM
    axial back pain, 135
    neurological deficits, 136
    orthopedic deformity, 136
    postoperative recurrence of symptoms
        missed secondary tethering lesion, 136–137
        regrowth of spur, 137

retethering, 137
    urological symptoms, 136
Lumbar SCMs, 103

M
Meningocele, 141
Meningomyeloceles (MMC), 37, 101, 141
Meninx primitiva cells, 12
Meninx primitiva precursor cells, 3
Midline axial integration during gastrulation, 12
Midline bone septum resection, surgical technique
    of, 35
Midline osseocartilaginous septum, 53
Midline septum development, 53–54
Multicomponent complex spinal dysraphism,
    103–104
Multilevel complex spinal dysraphism, 104
Muscle charting, 124
Myelocystocele (MMC), 21–22, 104
Myelomeningoceles, 12

N
Neural tube defects (NTDs)
    anesthetic concerns in patients with, 149*t*
        airway and respiratory evaluation, 142
        choice of anesthetic agents, 146
        fasting guidelines for pediatric patients, 143*t*
        induction of general anesthesia, 144–145
        intraoperative blood transfusion, 147
        intraoperative fluid management, 145–146
        intraoperative systemic complications,
            147–148
        latex sensitivity, 143
        OT preparation, 144
        perioperative investigations, 142–143
        postoperative care, 148
        preanesthetic evaluation, 141
        preanesthetic preparation, 143
        in prone position, 146*f*
        reversal, 148
        systemic evaluation, 141–142
    cellular mechanisms causing, 14
    definition of, 141
    embryogenesis of, 12–14
    genetic cause for, 13
    incidence of, 13
    open and closed, 141
    retrospective interpretation of, 13*f*
Neural tube formation, 10–11
Neurenteric canal formation, 10, 11*f*
Neurocutaneous markers, 25
Neuroectoderm, 10
Neurological deficits, 136
Neurological injury, 129–130
Neuromonitoring, 129
Notochord formation, 10–12
    fusion with endoderm, 10
    neural tube formation, 10–11
    neurenteric canal formation, 10, 11*f*

secondary neurulation, 11–12
spinal neurocele occlusion, 12

O
Occult spinal dysraphism, 17
OEIS complex, 105
Orthopedic deformity, 136
Osseocartilaginous tissue, 4
Osseous/fibrous-cartilaginous septum, 64
OT preparation, 144

P
Pang's unified theory of embryogenesis, 3
Passive warming devices, 144
Perioperative investigations, 142–143
Postoperative care, 129, 148
Postoperative recurrence of symptoms
    missed secondary tethering lesion, 136–137
    regrowth of spur, 137
    retethering, 137
Preanesthetic evaluation, 141
Preanesthetic preparation, 143
Primary SCM/occult SC SCM type I, 23–24, 24*f*
Primitive streak, 9
Prophylactic surgery, in SCM, 113, 115–116
Pseudomeningocele, 130

R
Regrowth of spur, 137
Renal function tests, 123
Retethering, 130, 137
Reversal of anesthesia, 148

S
Scoliosis management, 37, 115
Secondary neurulation, 11–12
Secondary tethering lesion, missed, 136–137
Septum, division of, 128
Spinal cord dysraphism, 25
Spinal dysraphisms
    cliniconeuroradiological classification for, 101
    congenital malformations, 21
    open form of, 21
    SCMs associated with, 21–22
Spinal neurocele occlusion, 12
Split cord malformations (SCM), 113
    anatomy of, 31–32
    associated anomalies with, 25*t*
    associated with spinal/cranial dysraphisms,
        21–22
    characterization of, 17
    classification of, 31–32, 63–64, 121, 122*f*, 122*t*,
        135
    clinical features, 4, 17, 25–26
    clinical presentation, 113–114, 121
    common location of, 113
    completeness of spur, 21
    complications
        CSF leak, 129

neurological injury, 129–130
        pseudomeningocele, 130
        retethering, 130
        surgical site infections, 130
    composite, 19–20, 20*f*, 102
        cases of, 83–84
        clinical findings, 84
        clinical significance, 83
        complex spinal dysraphic abnormality in, 81
        distribution of spurs in, 83
        embryogenesis, 82
        incidence of, 82, 102
        single stage surgery for, 84–85
    cord segments, 12
    definition, 9
    diagnostic imaging, 4, 26
    embryogenesis, 3–4, 24–25, 53
        gastrulation, 9–10
        notochord formation, 10–12
        SCM type I, 12
        unified theory on, 12, 53–54
    etiopathogenesis, 53
    fore- and midgut anomalies associated with, 3
    hypotheses for genesis of, 3
    inheritance, 32
    location of spur, 20
    long-term outcome of, 135–137
    with low-lying cord, management plan of, 115*t*
    management, 4–5
        algorithm, 130
        indications, 124
        neuromonitoring, 129
        preoperative preparation, 124
        surgical procedure, 125–129
    midline osseocartilaginous septum, 53
    morphology of, 3
    myelocystocele, 21–22
    numbers of spur, 21
    pathogenesis of, 9
    postoperative care, 129
    prophylactic surgery in (*See* Prophylactic
        surgery, in SCM)
    radiological workup, 4
    subclassification of, 3
    treatment and outcome, 26–27, 114–115
    type III SCMs, 21
    type II SCM (*See* Type II SCM)
    type I SCM (*See* Type I SCM)
Spur
    with intracranial/extracranial malformations,
        23
    regrowth of, 137
Surgical management of SCM. *See also* Prophylactic
    surgery, in SCM
    long-term outcomes of (*See* Long-term
        outcomes of SCM)
    surgery for cervical SCMs
        complications, 74–75
        indications for, 73

IONM, 73
  laminoplasty, 74
  laminotomy, 73–74
  outcome, 74
  pedicle screw fixation, 74
  surgery for type II SCM
    division of septum, 128
    filum terminale transection, 129
    laminectomy/laminotomy, 128
  surgery for type I SCM
    intradural pathologies and, 128
    lamiectomy and isolation of spur, 126–127
    unification of dural sacs, 128
Surgical site infections, 130
Systemic evaluation, 141–142

T
Teratogenic effect and neural tube defects, 14
Terminal myelocystocele, 104
Tethering elements, in SCM type II, 47
Type II SCM, 3, 9, 17, 43
  clinical presentation, 45–46
  diagnostic imaging, 46–47
  embryogenesis and histopathology, 43–45
  investigations, 114, 122–123
  management, 47–48
  radiological workup for, 46–47
  surgery for, 128–129
    division of septum, 128
    filum terminale transection, 129

  laminectomy/laminotomy, 128
Type I SCM, 3, 9, 17, 18*f*, 19*f*, 22, 43, 81
  anatomy, 31
  clinical presentation, 31–34
  complications, 36
  imaging, 34–35
  inheritance, 32
  investigations, 114, 122–123
  management, 35–36
    outcome, 37
    postoperative care, 36
    scoliosis, 37
    surgical technique, 35–36
    timing of surgery, 35
  subclassification for, 23–24, 24*f*, 31–32, 121–122, 122*f*, 122*t*
  surgery for, 126
    intradural pathologies and, 128
    lamiectomy and isolation of spur, 126–127
    unification of dural sacs, 128

U
Ultrasonography (USG), 123
Unification of dural sacs, 128
Unified theory of embryogenesis, 12, 53–54
Urodynamic studies (UDS), 123
Urological symptoms, 136

V
Ventral septa, 48